L[illegible] Science

T0253538

Vol. [illegible] Automata, Languages and Programming. [illegible] Edited by [illegible] IX, 5[illegible] pages. 1986.

Vol. [illegible] [illegible] pages. 1986.

Vol. [illegible] Advances in Cryptology – Proceedings of CRYPTO '84. Edited by G.R. Blakley and D. Chaum. IX, 4[illegible] pages. 1985.

Vol. [illegible] Proceedings. [illegible] D. Brookes, A.W. [illegible] pages. 1985.

Vol. [illegible] [illegible] 1985.

Vol. 199: Fundamentals of Computation Theory. Proceedings, 1985. Edited by L. Budach. XII, 533 pages. 1985.

Vol. 200: [illegible] VI, [illegible] pages. 1985.

Vol. 201: Functional Programming Languages and Computer Architecture. Proceedings, 1985. Edited by J.-P. Jouannaud. VI, 413 pages. 1985.

Vol. [illegible] Rewriting Techniques and Applications. Edited by J.-P. Jouannaud. [illegible] pages. 1985.

Vol. [illegible] EUROCAL '85. Proceedings Vol. 1, 1985. Edited by B. Buchberger. [illegible] 1985.

Vol. 20[illegible] [illegible]

Vol. [illegible] [illegible] Proceedings, 1985. Edited by [illegible] 1985.

Vol. [illegible] Proceedings, 1986. Edited by [illegible] pages. 1986.

Vol. [illegible] [illegible] pages. 1986.

Vol. [illegible] [illegible] Proceedings, 1985. Edited by [illegible] pages. 1986.

Vol. [illegible] Current Trends in Concurrency. Overviews and Tutorials. Edited by J.W. de Bakker, W.-P. de Roever and G. Rozenberg. [illegible] pages. 1986.

Vol. 225: Third International Conference on Logic Programming. Proceedings, 1986. Edited by E. Shapiro. IX, 720 pages. 1986.

Vol. 226: Automata, Languages and Programming. Proceedings, 1986. Edited by L. Kott. IX, 474 pages. 1986.

Vol. 227: VLSI Algorithms and Architectures – AWOC 86. Proceedings, 1986. Edited by F. Makedon, K. Mehlhorn, T. Papatheodorou and P. Spirakis. VIII, 328 pages. 1986.

Vol. 228: Applied Algebra, Algorithmics and Error-Correcting Codes. AAECC-2. Proceedings, 1984. Edited by A. Poli. VI, 265 pages. 1986.

Vol. 229: Algebraic Algorithms and Error-Correcting Codes. AAECC-3. Proceedings, 1985. Edited by J. Calmet. VII, 416 pages. 1986.

Vol. [illegible] [illegible]

Vol. [illegible] [illegible] 1986.

Lecture Notes in Computer Science

Vol. 192: Automata on Infinite Words. Proceedings, 1984. Edited by M. Nivat and D. Perrin. V, 216 pages.1985.

Vol. 193: Logics of Programs. Proceedings, 1985. Edited by R. Parikh. VI, 424 pages. 1985.

Vol. 194: Automata, Languages and Programming. Proceedings, 1985. Edited by W. Brauer. IX, 520 pages. 1985.

Vol. 195: H. J. Stüttgen, A Hierarchical Associative Processing System. XII, 273 pages. 1985.

Vol. 196: Advances in Cryptology. Proceedings of CRYPTO '84. Edited by G. R. Blakley and D. Chaum. IX, 491 pages.1985.

Vol. 197: Seminar on Concurrency. Proceedings, 1984. Edited by S. D. Brookes, A. W. Roscoe and G. Winskel. X, 523 pages. 1985.

Vol. 198: A. Businger, PORTAL Language Description. VIII, 186 pages. 1985.

Vol. 199: Fundamentals of Computation Theory. Proceedings, 1985. Edited by L. Budach. XII, 533 pages. 1985.

Vol. 200: J. L. A. van de Snepscheut, Trace Theory and VLSI Design. VI, 0–140 pages. 1985.

Vol. 201: Functional Programming Languages and Computer Architecture. Proceedings, 1985. Edited by J.-P. Jouannaud. VI, 413 pages. 1985.

Vol. 202: Rewriting Techniques and Applications. Edited by J.-P. Jouannaud. VI, 441 pages. 1985.

Vol. 203: EUROCAL '85. Proceedings Vol. 1, 1985. Edited by B. Buchberger. V, 233 pages. 1985.

Vol. 204: EUROCAL '85. Proceedings Vol. 2, 1985. Edited by B. F. Caviness. XVI, 650 pages. 1985.

Vol. 205: P. Klint, A Study in String Processing Languages. VIII, 165 pages. 1985.

Vol. 206: Foundations of Software Technology and Theoretical Computer Science. Proceedings, 1985. Edited by S.N. Maheshwari. IX, 522 pages. 1985.

Vol. 207: The Analysis of Concurrent Systems. Proceedings, 1983. Edited by B.T. Denvir, W.T. Harwood, M.I. Jackson and M.J. Wray. VII, 398 pages. 1985.

Vol. 208: Computation Theory. Proceedings, 1984. Edited by A. Skowron. VII, 397 pages. 1985.

Vol. 209: Advances in Cryptology. Proceedings of EUROCRYPT '84. Edited by T. Beth, N. Cot and I. Ingemarsson. VII, 491 pages. 1985.

Vol. 210: STACS 86. Proceedings, 1986. Edited by B. Monien and G. Vidal-Naquet. IX, 368 pages. 1986.

Vol. 211: U. Schöning, Complexity and Structure. V, 99 pages. 1986.

Vol. 212: Interval Mathematics 1985. Proceedings, 1985. Edited by K. Nickel. VI, 227 pages. 1986.

Vol. 213: ESOP 86. Proceedings, 1986. Edited by B. Robinet and R. Wilhelm. VI, 374 pages. 1986.

Vol. 214: CAAP '86. 11th Colloquium on Trees in Algebra and Programming. Proceedings, 1986. Edited by P. Franchi-Zannettacci. VI, 306 pages. 1986.

Vol. 215: Mathematical Methods of Specification and Synthesis of Software Systems '85. Proceedings, 1985. Edited by W. Bibel and K.P. Jantke. 245 pages. 1986.

Vol. 216: Ch. Fernstrom, I. Kruzela, B. Svensson, LUCAS Associative Array Processor: Design, Programming and Application Studies. XII, 323 pages. 1986.

Vol. 217: Programs as Data Objects. Proceedings, 1985. Edited by H. Ganzinger and N.D. Jones. X, 324 pages. 1986.

Vol. 218: Advances in Cryptology – CRYPTO '85. Proceedings, 1985. Edited by H.C. Williams. X, 548 pages. 1986.

Vol. 219: Advances in Cryptology – EUROCRYPT '85. Proceedings, 1985. Edited by F. Pichler. IX, 281 pages. 1986.

Vol. 220: RIMS Symposia on Software Science and Engineering II. Proceedings, 1983 and 1984. Edited by E. Goto, K. Araki and T. Yuasa. XI, 323 pages. 1986.

Vol. 221: Logic Programming '85. Proceedings, 1985. Edited by E. Wada. IX, 311 pages. 1986.

Vol. 222: Advances in Petri Nets 1985. Edited by G. Rozenberg. VI, 498 pages. 1986.

Vol. 223: Structure in Complexity Theory. Proceedings, 1986. Edited by A.L. Selman. VI, 401 pages. 1986.

Vol. 224: Current Trends in Concurrency. Overviews and Tutorials. Edited by J.W. de Bakker, W.-P. de Roever and G. Rozenberg. XII, 716 pages. 1986.

Vol. 225: Third International Conference on Logic Programming. Proceedings, 1986. Edited by E. Shapiro. IX, 720 pages. 1986.

Vol. 226: Automata, Languages and Programming. Proceedings, 1986. Edited by L. Kott. IX, 474 pages. 1986.

Vol. 227: VLSI Algorithms and Architectures – AWOC 86. Proceedings, 1986. Edited by F. Makedon, K. Mehlhorn, T. Papatheodorou and P. Spirakis. VIII, 328 pages. 1986.

Vol. 228: Applied Algebra, Algorithmics and Error-Correcting Codes. AAECC-2. Proceedings, 1984. Edited by A. Poli. VI, 265 pages. 1986.

Vol. 229: Algebraic Algorithms and Error-Correcting Codes. AAECC-3. Proceedings, 1985. Edited by J. Calmet. VII, 416 pages. 1986.

Vol. 230: 8th International Conference on Automated Deduction. Proceedings, 1986. Edited by J.H. Siekmann. X, 708 pages. 1986.

Vol. 231: R. Hausser, NEWCAT: Parsing Natural Language Using Left-Associative Grammar. II, 540 pages. 1986.

Vol. 232: Fundamentals of Artificial Intelligence. Edited by W. Bibel and Ph. Jorrand. VII, 313 pages. 1986.

Vol. 233: Mathematical Foundations of Computer Science 1986. Proceedings, 1986. Edited by J. Gruska, B. Rovan and J. Wiedermann. IX, 650 pages. 1986.

Vol. 234: Concepts in User Interfaces: A Reference Model for Command and Response Languages. By Members of IFIP Working Group 2.7. Edited by D. Beech. X, 116 pages. 1986.

Vol. 235: Accurate Scientific Computations. Proceedings, 1985. Edited by W.L. Miranker and R.A. Toupin. XIII, 205 pages. 1986.

Vol. 236: TEX for Scientific Documentation. Proceedings, 1986. Edited by J. Désarménien. VI, 204 pages. 1986.

Vol. 237: CONPAR 86. Proceedings, 1986. Edited by W. Händler, D. Haupt, R. Jeltsch, W. Juling and O. Lange. X, 418 pages. 1986.

Vol. 238: L. Naish, Negation and Control in Prolog. IX, 119 pages. 1986.

Vol. 239: Mathematical Foundations of Programming Semantics. Proceedings, 1985. Edited by A. Melton. VI, 395 pages. 1986.

Vol. 240: Category Theory and Computer Programming. Proceedings, 1985. Edited by D. Pitt, S. Abramsky, A. Poigné and D. Rydeheard. VII, 519 pages. 1986.

Vol. 241: Foundations of Software Technology and Theoretical Computer Science. Proceedings, 1986. Edited by K.V. Nori. XII, 519 pages. 1986.

Vol. 242: Combinators and Functional Programming Languages. Proceedings, 1985. Edited by G. Cousineau, P.-L. Curien and B. Robinet. V, 208 pages. 1986.

Vol. 243: ICDT '86. Proceedings, 1986. Edited by G. Ausiello and P. Atzeni. VI, 444 pages. 1986.

Vol. 244: Advanced Programming Environments. Proceedings, 1986. Edited by R. Conradi, T.M. Didriksen and D.H. Wanvik. VII, 604 pages. 1986

Lecture Notes in Computer Science

Edited by G. Goos and J. Hartmanis

281

Alica Kelemenová Jozef Kelemen (Eds.)

Trends, Techniques, and Problems in Theoretical Computer Science

4th International Meeting of Young Computer Scientists
Smolenice, Czechoslovakia, October 13–17, 1986
Selected Contributions

Springer-Verlag
Berlin Heidelberg New York London Paris Tokyo

Editors

Alica Kelemenová
Mathematical Institute, Slovak Academy of Sciences
Obrancov mieru 49, 814 73 Bratislava, Czechoslovakia

Jozef Kelemen
Institute of Computer Science, Comenius University
Mlynská dolina, 842 43 Bratislava, Czechoslovakia

CR Subject Classification (1987): A.0, A.1, F.1.1, F.1.3, F.4.1–3, I.2.1, I.2.4

ISBN 3-540-18535-6 Springer-Verlag Berlin Heidelberg New York
ISBN 0-387-18535-6 Springer-Verlag New York Berlin Heidelberg

Printed in Germany

Printing and binding: Druckhaus Beltz, Hemsbach/Bergstr.
2145/3140-543210

Foreword

This volume contains the written versions of selected contributions from the scientific programme of the **Fourth International Meeting of Young Computer Scientists** held at Smolenice Castle (Czechoslovakia), October 13-17, 1986.

Organized biennially since 1980, the meetings are intended to stimulate the scientific activity of beginners in computer science, mainly that of both university students in the final years of their studies and of graduates. Therefore, the scientific programme of the meetings include tutorials and more invited lectures than it is usual at conferences. Participants have the possibility to submit papers and to present their scientific results during the meetings, and to gain the first experience in the work of scientific meetings, as well as to gain an insight into contemporary trends, techniques, and problems of theoretical computer science and related fields.

In the present volume the texts of the tutorial of IMYCS'86 as well as the texts of all invited talks are included together with some selected short communications presented during the meeting's regular and informal evening sessions.

Thematically, the volume is divided into four chapters. Within each chapter the contributions are ordered alphabetically according to the authors' names.

In the first chapter papers devoted to the study of VLSI algorithms (J. Hromkovič), and to problems of formal language theory (J. Karhumäki, J. Sakarovitch, and Z. Tuza) are included.

The second chapter contains a communication by E. Csuhaj-Varjú and invited lectures by H. C. M. Kleijn and G. Păun dealing with various aspects of the theory of formal grammars.

Contributions in the third chapter deal with two biologically motivated formalisms: homogeneous structures (in the contribution by V. Aladyev) and L-systems in the texts of the IMYCS'86 tutorial delivered by A. Lindenmayer, and in the short communication by M. Kráľová.

The fourth chapter is devoted to some (rather) theoretical topics of Artificial Intelligence, particularly to problems concerning the formal treatment of knowledge bases (in the contribution by I. Kalaš), to automation of hypotheses formation (in the invited paper by F. N. Springsteel), and to new perspectives of logic programming (in the invited paper by P. Szeredi).

We are indebted to all the contributors to this volume for their cooperation. Also we would like to express our gratitude to Prof. Arto Salomaa for supporting our idea to publish this selection, and to the Springer-Verlag for helping us to realize it.

Bratislava, August 1987

Alica Kelemenová
Jozef Kelemen

CONTENTS

Chapter 1

VLSI AND FORMAL LANGUAGES

LOWER BOUND TECHNIQUES FOR VLSI ALGORITHMS

Juraj Hromkovič [+]
Department of Theoretical Cybernetics, Comenius University
842 15 Bratislava, Czechoslovakia

1. INTRODUCTION

The basic concept of complexity theory for VLSI was given by Thompson [41,42]. Since hundreds of papers dealing with VLSI algorithms were published in the last seven years we have no chance to consider all of them. The aim of this paper is to outline an short overview involving the basic concepts in the proving of lower bounds for A, AT, and AT^2 complexity measures of VLSI algorithms, the new approaches making the lower bound proof technique more successful, and the use of the idea of "information transfer" for VLSI for the obtaining of lower bounds on different complexity measures of another computing models. This survey is supplemented by some new ideas and results which can be useful in proving lower bounds for some special VLSI models. In the case that the reader is interested in other questions concerning VLSI theory too, the monograph of Ullman |43| is much recommended.

This paper consists of 8 sections. Section 2 involves the basic definitions covering the definition of VLSI circuits. Motivated by the fact that VLSI circuits were not described as mathematical structures till now (the usual definitions of VLSI circuit are speaking about a circuit with a number of some properties described in an informal way) we give the definition of VLSI circuits in this way. Adding to this model some futher requirements related to the current technology one can obtain definitions of several special models. Section 3 and Section 4 resp. involves the outline of lower bound techniques for the complexity measure A and AT respectively. A generalization of the technique for proving lower bounds on the most studied complexity measure AT^2 is presented in Section 5. Some application of this technique based on

---

+ This work was partially supported by the ŠPZV$_I$II-8-1/10 grant and the Computer Science Institute of Comenius University.

"information transfer" are shown in Section 6. A short survey of basic results concerning the communication complexity model that represents an absraction of information transfer in VLSI circuit is given in Section 7. Section 8 consists of some examples showing that the concept of communication complexity can be used to obtain lower bounds on different complexity measures of other computing models.

2. DEFINITIONS

The aim of this section is to give the formal definition of VLSI circuits. Before we do it we make precise the notion of problem considered here.

Definition 2.1 Let $X=\{x_1,\dots,x_n\}$, $Y=\{y_1,\dots,y_m\}$ be the sets of Boolean variables. A problem instance P from the input variables X to the output variables Y is a set of Boolean functions $\{f_1,f_2,\dots,f_m\}$ such that $f_i: X\to\{0,1\}$ and $y_i=f_i(x_1,x_2,\dots,x_n)$ for $i=1,\dots,m$. The positive integer n is called the size of P.

Definition 2.2 A problem is an infinite sequence of problem instances, where each two instances in the sequence have a different size parameter n.

An example of a problem can be the recognition of a language $L\subseteq\{0,1\}^*$. To see this fact we associate with each language $L\subseteq\{0,1\}^*$ the infinite sequence of Boolean functions $\{h_i^L\}_{i=1}$, where $h_i^L: \{0,1\}^i \to \{0,1\}$ and $h_i^L(x_1,\dots,x_i)=1$ iff $x_1x_2\dots x_i \in L\cap\{0,1\}^i$. So, the i-th problem instance is the Boolean function h_i^L.

Another example can be the problem of sorting n numbers coded binary in the words of fixed length m. Clearly, for each positive integer n, we have a problem instance from input variables $X= x_1,x_2,\dots$ $\dots,x_{mn}$ to output variables $Y= y_1,y_2,\dots,y_{mn}$ as a set of mn Boolean functions.

Definition 2.3 A 4-graph is a directed graph $G=(V,E)$ with the property that, for each $v\in V$, the sum of edges outputing from v and inputing to v is bounded by 4.

Definition 2.4 A VLSI graph M_G is a 4-graph G embeded in the lattice in such a way that each square of the lattice has one of the following contentses:

(a) an vertex of the graph,

(b) an directed line going in the horisontal or in the vertical direction (this line is a part of an edge of the graph),

(c) one broken line coming in the lattice square in one of two vertical (horisontal) directions and outcoming in one of two horisontal (vertical) directions,

(d) two crossing lines, one going in the horisontal direction, the other in the vertical direction (this depicts the place of two crossing edges without any vertex of the embeding of the directed graph in the plane),

(e) the empty contents.

The VLSI graph M_G is called the embeding of G in the lattice too.

Definition 2.5 The area complexity of an VLSI graph is the area of a minimal rectangler involving all non-empty squares of the lattice. The area complexity of a 4-graph G is the minimum of area complexities of all VLSI graphs which are embedings of G in the lattice.

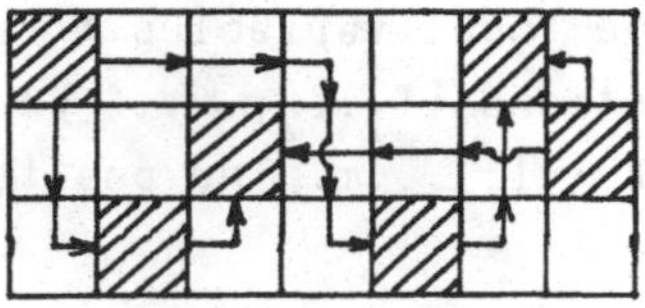

Fig.1

To see an example of a VLSI graph we give Fig.1. One can find all possible contentses of the lattice squares in Fig.1. The space complexity of this VLSI graph is 3 x 7 = 21 . The full lattice squares represents the vertices of the graph.

Definition 2.6 A VLSI circuit is a 6-tuple $R=\langle M_G,P,p,X,Y,r\rangle$, where:

(1) M_G is a VLSI graph that is the embeding of a 4-graph $G=(V,E)$ in the lattice.

(2) P is a finite, nonempty set (called processor set) of functions from $\{0,1\}^i$ to $\{0,1\}^j$, where $i+j \leq 4$, $i,j \in \{0,1,2,3,4\}$.

(3) p is a function from V to P such that, for each $v \in V$ with the indegree i and the outdegree j $p(v)=f_v$, where f_v: $\{0,1\}^i \rightarrow \{0,1\}^j$.

(4) $X=\{x_1,\ldots,x_n\}$ is the set of input variables.

(5) $Y=\{y_1,\ldots,y_m\}$ is the set of output variables.

(6) r is a function (called input/output function) from $X \cup Y$ to $V \times N$ such that for all $x,y \in X$ (Y) , $x \neq y$, $r(x) \neq r(y)$ holds, and if $(v,t) = r(x)$ for a $x \in X$ (Y) then v is called the input (output) processor, and v has indegree (outdegree) zero and outdegree (indegree) at most three.

Definition 2.7 A VLSI circuit $R = \langle M_G,P,p,X,Y,r\rangle$ is called B-circuit when, for all $v \in V$ such that $(v,t)=r(x)$ for some $x \in X \cup Y$, v is laid on the border of M_G. For a positive integer k , a VLSI circuit (B-circuit) R is called kVLSI circuit (kB-circuit) when for all $v \in V$ there sre at most k input variables $x \in X$ such that $r(x)=(v,t)$ for some $t \in N$. A B-circuit (kB-circuit) R is called <u>B(i,j)-circuit</u> (<u>kB(i,j)-circuit</u>) if R has i borders involving all input processors and no output processor, and j borders involving all output processors.

We have introduced formal definitions of different models of VLSI circuits that were usually defined only informally |41-43|. The computation of a VLSI circuit can be defined as follows. Let $R = \langle M_G, P, p, X, Y, r \rangle$ with $G=(V,E)$ be a VLSI circuit, and let $v_1, \ldots v_m$ be a fixed order of all vertices in V. Let $e_{i1}, \ldots, e_{ij_i}$, for $j_i \in \{1,2,3,4\}$, be the sequence of all input edges of v_i from E for all v_i's that are not input processors, and let e_{i1} be the input edge of v_i (not in E) if v_i is an input processor. For each time unit t one can associate a Boolean value a^t_{ik} to each e_{ik}, $i \in \{1,\ldots,m\}$, $k \in \{1,\ldots,j_i\}$. In the time unit $t=0$ all input edges from E have the value 0. For all $x \in X$, if $r(x)=(v_i,0)$ then e_{i1} has the value of the input variable x, if for all x assigned to v_i $r(x)=(v_i,t')$, for a $t' \neq 0$, then e_{i1} has the value 0. Clearly, knowing the values of all input edges in the time unit t we obtain the input values in the time unit t+1 as output values of all (vertices) processors with given inputs. The input edge of an input processor v has in the time unit t either the value 0 (if no input variable is coming in v in the time unit t) or the value of an input variable coming in v in the time unit t.

We define a <u>state</u> s_t of the VLSI circuit R in the time unit t as the sequence $a^t_{i1},\ldots,a^t_{ij_1},a^t_{i2},\ldots,a^t_{ij_2},\ldots,a^t_{im},\ldots,a^t_{ij_m}$ of values of the input edges $e_{i1},\ldots,e_{ij_1},e_{i2},\ldots,e_{ij_2},\ldots,e_{im},\ldots e_{ij_m}$. A <u>computation</u> of the VLSI circuit R on an input vector **a** is a sequence of states $S_0, S_1, \ldots, S_t, S_{t+1}, \ldots$ such that for each t S_t is the state of R working on input **a** in the time unit t. Taking the output values of output processors in the time unit determined by r one can associate exactly one problem instance to R.

<u>Definition 2.8</u> The <u>time complexity T(R)</u> of a VLSI circuit $R = \langle M_G, P, p, X, Y, r \rangle$ is $\max\{t \mid (v,t)=r(y) \text{ for a } y \in Y\}$.

In the case that we have an infinite sequence of VLSI circuits solving a problem we can consider the area and time complexity as functions of the size of the problem. For an infinite sequence of VLSI circuits **R** we denote by the function from positive integers to positive integers $T_{\mathbf{R}}(n)$ ($A_{\mathbf{R}}(n)$) the <u>time</u> (<u>area</u>) <u>complexity</u> of **R**.

Now, let us define the area and time complexity of a problem.

<u>Definition 2.9</u> Let $\mathbf{P} = \{P_i\}_{i=1}^{\infty}$ be a problem, and let n_i be the size of the problem instance P_i for any $i=1,2,\ldots$. Let, for $i=1,2,\ldots$,

R_i be a circuit solving P_i with minimal area (time, area·time, area·(time)^2) complexity. We say that the <u>area</u> (<u>time</u>, <u>area·time</u>, <u>area·(time)^2</u>) <u>complexity of P</u> is the function A_P (T_P, AT_P, AT_P^2) from $\{n_i \mid i=1,2,\ldots\}$ to positive integers defined by $A_P(n_i) = A(R_i)$ ($T_P(n_i) = T(R_i)$, $AT_P(n_i) = A(R_i)T(R_i)$, $AT_P^2(n_i) = A(R_i)(T(R_i))^{2^i}$) for all positive integers i .

We note that the circuits solving the same problem instance with minimal area, time, or area(time)^2 complexity can be very different. It follows from the fact that a decrease of the area complexity can be compensated by an increase of the time complexity and vice versa. So, to investigate only the area (time) complexity of a problem **P** without considering its time (area) complexity grants no sufficient information about the hardness of P . Realizing this fact one study mostly the area-time tradeoffs of problems.

3. LOWER BOUNDS ON AREA

The area of a VLSI circuit solving a specific problem was investigated in several papers (see, for example, |4,6,10,13,19,26,27, 39|). The reason to deal with the area complexity measure follows from the technology. If one is able to produce a good, special chip of the area complexity A with a probability p (for example, if p=1/10 then it means that 10% of the produced chips are good) then the probability of producing a good chip of area complexity 2A is p^2 (1% in our example). So, the charge of the VLSI chips growths exponentially with the area complexity of these chips.

The obtaining of lower bounds on the area of VLSI circuits is based on the following fact. Each circuit having area A cannot remember more than 3A/2 bits in its state from one time unit to the next one. Following this we are formulating a general "algorithm" for proving lower bounds on area of VLSI circuits computing specific problems.

" A-algorithm"

Input: A problem instance P with the set of input variables X and the set of output variables Y .

Step1: Prove, for a $X_1 \subseteq X$ and $Y_1 \subseteq Y$, that there is a time unit t such that all input variables from X_1 have to be read before the time unit t , and all output variables from Y_1 have to be computed after the time unit t in any VLSI circuit solving P .

Step 2: Prove, for a number d, that there are d different assignments of values to the input variables from X_1 which require distinct assignments of values to the output variables from Y_1 .

Output: $3A \geq 2\log_2 d$

The correctness of "A-algorithm" follows from the fact that the VLSI circuit that is in the same state in the same time unit t for two different inputs (differing only in the values of the variables from X_1) cannot distinguish between these two inputs, and has to compute the same values for all output variables computed after the time unit t .

Using "A-algorithm" one can provide, for example, that the sorting of m digits of the length $|\log_2 m| + 1$ in the binary coding requires $3A \geq 2m$ |43|.

We conclude this section with an interesting result obtained by Gubáš and Waczulík |13|. They have found two languages L_1 and L_2 that can be recognized by B-circuits having constant area complexity, but the language $L_1 \cup L_2$ require $\Omega(n^{1/2})$ area complexity to be recognized on general model of VLSI circuits.

4. LOWER BOUNDS ON THE TRADEOFF AT

There is a very simple lower bound proof technique for the complexity measure AT studied, for example, in |5,31-33,38,43|. It is based on the following theorem |43|.

<u>Theorem 4.1</u> Let P be a problem instance with the set of input variables X , and the set of output variables Y . Let $d = \max\{|X|, |Y|\}$. Then $AT \geq d$.

<u>Proof</u>: In each time unit the VLSI circuit can read (write) at most A bits.

Using Theorem 2.1 we have that $AT \geq m\log_2 m$ for any VLSI circuit sorting m numbers of the length $|\log_2 m| + 1$ in binary coding.

5. LOWER BOUNDS ON THE TRADEOFF AT^2

The complexity measure AT^2 is the most studied area-time tradeoff in VLSI theory |1-3,5,9,12-23,25,30,38,41-45|. Opposite the lower bounds on A and AT based on memory requirements the lower bounds on AT^2 are based on the requirements on information flow within the chip. The idea follows from the fact that if we can prove that a certain amount of information (bits) I must flow across a boundary cutting a circuit R across the shorter dimension of VLSI graph area then we obtain $T(R)(A(R))^{1/2} \geq I$, i.e. $T(R)^2 A(R) \geq I^2$.

First, let us present the original lower bound technique based on information transfer |1,3,5,9,12-17,25,30,38,41,42,44,45|. This original technique was the object of criticism in |2,18,43|. It led to a new definition of "information transfer" in |2| whose generalization related to the possibility of obtaining stronger lower bounds for special VLSI models is presented in the second part of this section.

The lower bound technique based on information transfer provides no higher lower bounds for AT^2 than $\Omega(n^2)$. So, the following theorem shows that it has no sense to study the information transfer of (n/c)VLSI circuits, where n is the size of a problem instance and c is a constant according to n.

<u>Theorem 5.1</u> Let c be a positive integer, and let $\mathbf{P} = \{P_i\}_{i=1}^{\infty}$ be a problem, where for each i the size of P_i is n_i and $\mathbf{P}_i$ depends on all its n_i input variables. Let $\mathbf{R} = \{R_i\}_{i=1}^{\infty}$ be a sequnce of VLSI circuits solving $\mathbf{P}$, where, for each i=1,2,... , R_i is no (n_i/c)VLSI circuit. Then $A_{\mathbf{R}}(n_i)T^2_{\mathbf{R}}(n_i) \geq (n_i)^2/c^2$.

<u>Proof</u>: Let, for any positive integer i, R_i is not an (n_i/c)VLSI circuit. It implies that R_i involves an input processor v assigned to at least $(n_i/c)+1$ input variables. Since P_i depends on all input variables R_i cannot give all output values before all input values were read. The processor v need at least (n_i/c) time units to read all input values of variables assigned to it which implies $T(R_i) \geq n_i/c$. So, for any positive integer i, $(T(R_i))^2 \geq n_i^2/c^2$, i.e. $T^2_{\mathbf{R}}(n_i) \geq n_i^2/c^2$.

Realizing the meaning of Theorem 5.1 one can simply seen that for building of lower bound technique based on information transfer it suffices to deal with kVLSI circuits only, where k is the size of the problem instance divided ba an arbitrarly large constant.

Now, let us outline the "strategy" for proving lower bounds on AT^2. To do it we need the following lemma.

<u>Lemma 5.2</u> Let $c \geq 3$ be a positive integer, and P be a problem instance with the set X of n input variables. Let R be an (n/c)VLSI circuit solving P. Then there is a line involving at most one single jog (see Fig.2) that divides the circuit R into two parts, each having assigned between $n - n/c$ and $n + n/c$ input variables.

<u>Proof</u>. The proof directly follows from the fact that there are at most

n/c input variables assigned to one processor. So, if we have a circuit divided into two parts and we take one square of the lattice from the

Figure 2:

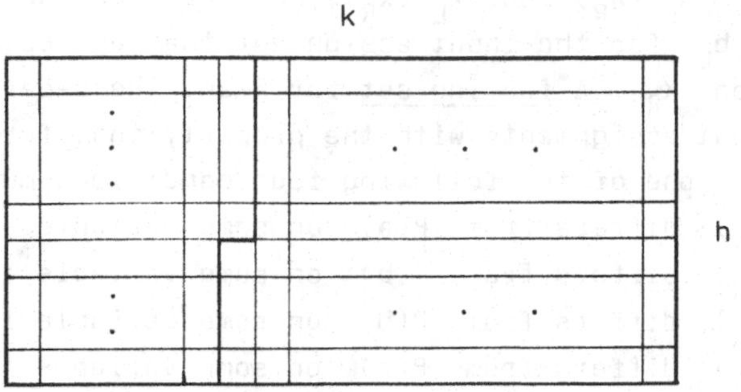

left side and we give it to the right side of the circuit then the number of input variables assigned to the left side is decreased at most by n/c input variables and the number of input variables assigned to the right side is increased at most by n/c input variables. Clearly, an algorithm finding the dividing line with at most one single jog can start with the square in upper-right corner and proceed adding one square after the other .

Now, the idea consists in proving that at least d bits must flow through the line depicted at Fig.2, for a positive integer d . Assuming withou loss of generality that $k \geq h$ we have $(h+1)T(R) \geq d$, i.e.

$$2A(R)(T(R))^2 \geq d^2 .$$

So, the problem of proving lower bound on AT^2 is transformed to proving "somethink" about information transfer of all circuits solving the problem instance considered. Now, let us make more precise what does this "somethink" mean.

<u>Definition 5.3</u> Let c be a positive integer, and let P_n be a problem instance with the set of input variables X, $|X|=n$, and the set of output variables Y . A <u>c-partition</u> for P_n is a 4-tuple (X_L, X_R, Y_L, Y_R) , where $X_L \cap X_R = Y_L \cap Y_R = \emptyset$, $X_L \cup X_R = X$, $n/2 - n/c \leq |X_L|, |X_R| \leq n/2 + n/c$, and $Y_L \cup Y_R = Y$.

Obviously, a partition can be assigned to each line dividing a circuit into two parts. Now, after defining the notion "fooling set" let us formulate the original "algorithm" used for proving lower bounds on AT^2 .

<u>Definition 5.4</u> Let c be a positive integer. Let $\mathbf{p}=(X_L, X_R, Y_L, Y_R)$ be a c-partition of a problem instance P of size n . An <u>input</u> (<u>output</u>) <u>assigment</u> for P is a mapping from X (Y) to $\{0,1\}$ giving a Boolean

value to each input (output) variable. For any input assignment **a** we denote by P(**a**) the output assignment to **a** (determined by P), and by $\mathbf{a}_L$ ($\mathbf{a}_R$) an input assignment from X_L (X_R) to $\{0,1\}$ such that **a** agree with $\mathbf{a}_L$ ($\mathbf{a}_R$) on X_L (X_R). For two input assignments **a** and **b** we use $\mathbf{a}_L\mathbf{b}_L$ for the input assignment that agrees with **a** on X_L and with **b** on X_R. A <u>fooling set</u> for P and the c-partition **p** is a set $\mathbf{A}_\mathbf{p}$ of input assignments with the property that for any distinct **a** and **b** in $\mathbf{A}_\mathbf{p}$, one of the following four conditions must hold.

1. $P(\mathbf{a}_L\mathbf{b}_R)$ differs from $P(\mathbf{a})$ on some variable in Y_L.
2. $P(\mathbf{a}_L\mathbf{b}_R)$ differs from $P(\mathbf{b})$ on some variable in Y_R.
3. $P(\mathbf{b}_L\mathbf{a}_R)$ differs from $P(\mathbf{b})$ on some variable in Y_L.
4. $P(\mathbf{b}_L\mathbf{a}_R)$ differs from $P(\mathbf{a})$ on some variable in Y_R.

" AT^2 original algorithm "

Input: A problem instance P.

Step1. Let $\mathbf{p}_1, \mathbf{p}_2, \dots \mathbf{p}_s$ be all different 3-partitions for P. Find, for each $i \in \{1,2,\dots,s\}$, $\mathbf{A}_i$ - the largest fooling set for $\mathbf{p}_i$.

Step2. Compute $d = \min\{\,|\mathbf{A}_i| \mid i=1,2,\dots,s\}$

Output: $9A(R)(T(R))^2 \geq (\log_2 d)^2$ for every VLSIcircuit R solving P.

What does imply the correctness of this algorithm ? It follows from the fact that, for any 3-partition **p** given by a line with at most one jog, the number of all different communications going through the line (a communication for a given input assignment is a sequence of all communication bits going through the line during the computation and ordered according to the time units (for one time unit the communication bits can be ordered , for example, according to the wires from up to down)) has to be greater than the size of largest fooling set for **p**. If not then there are two different assignments of values **a** and **b** from a fooling set **A** having the same communication. Clearly, the same communication for **a** and **b** implies:

a, $P(\mathbf{a}_L\mathbf{b}_R)$ agrees with $P(\mathbf{a})=P(\mathbf{a}_L\mathbf{a}_R)$ on all inpit variables in Y_L (because the same communication is going from the right side to the left side for both $\mathbf{a}_R$ and $\mathbf{b}_R$ on the right side whenever $\mathbf{a}_L$ is on the left side) ,

b, $P(\mathbf{a}_L\mathbf{b}_R)$ agrees with $P(\mathbf{b})$ on all variables in Y_R ,

c, $P(\mathbf{b}_L\mathbf{a}_R)$ agrees with $P(\mathbf{b})$ on all variables in Y_L ,

d, $P(\mathbf{b}_L\mathbf{a}_R)$ agrees with $P(\mathbf{a})$ on all variables in Y_R ,

which contradicts to the fact that **a** and **b** belongs to the fooling set **A** .

The technique introduced in the previous section was the object of criticism in |2,18| from the following two reasons:

i, There are very hard problems according to AT^2 which can be solved with small "information transfer".

ii, It is very hard to prove a high lower bound on "information transfer" as the minimum over all partitions of input variables. It holds in the cases too, where it seems to be obvious that a large information transfer is required.

The background of the drawbacks i, and ii, lays really in the fact that we do not need to take minimum of the sizes of fooling sets over all c-partitions, for some c. We try to illustrate it on the following example.

Let us have a problem consisting of a constant number of subproblems with disjoint sets of input variables. Let some of these subproblems require linear (maximal) information transfer, and let a small (constant) information transfer suffices to obtain the solution of the problem in the case that the solutions of the subproblems are known. Then, if we take a partition of the input bits that gives the input variables of some subproblems to the left part of the circuits, and the input variables of additional subproblems to the right side of the circuits, the problem can be solved with small (constant) information transfer. On the other hand the solution of the problem can require $AT^2 \in \Omega(n^2)$. In |2,15,18| it is shown how a problem with zero information transfer can be constructed from a problem with linear linear information transfer without decreasing the complexity AT^2 .

The drawbacks introduced above can be overwied choosing a subset Z of the set of input variables X and considering the partition of X as defined in what follows |2|.

<u>Definition 5.5</u> Let c be a positive integer, and let P be a problem instance with the set of input variables X , $|X| = n$, and the set of output variables Y . Let Z be a subset of X . A <u>c-partition for P according to Z</u> is a 5-tuple (Z, X_L, X_R, Y_L, Y_R) , where $X_L \cap X_R = Y_L \cap Y_R = \emptyset$, $X_L \cup X_R = X$, $Y_L \cup Y_R = Y$, and $|Z|/2 - |Z|/2c \leq |X_L \cap Z|, |X_R \cap Z| \leq |Z|/2 + |Z|/2c$.

It is no doubt that we can choose a line dividing the circuit into two parts such that at least $|Z|/2 - |Z|/2c$ input variables from Z are assigned to each side because we give no requirement on the partitioning of the input variables from $X-Z$ (for example, all input variables from $X-Z$ can be assigned to one side of the circuit).

Now, let us give the generalization of the notion "information content of P" for any problem P.

<u>Definition 5.6</u> Let $P = \{P_i\}_{i=1}^{\infty}$ be a problem and, for any $i \in N$, P_i be a problem instance with the set of input variables X_i, $|X_i|=i$, and the set of output variables Y_i. Let $c \geq 3$ be a positive integer and let **p** be a c-partition for P_i according to a $Z \subseteq X_i$. Define $I_c(P_i,\mathbf{p})$ to be the logarithm, base two, of the size of the largest fooling set for P_i and **p**. Let ç be a condition for **p** that can be considered as a property of some partitions. Let $M_c(Z)$ be the set off all c-partitions for P_i according to Z and let $M_c(Z,ç)) = \{\mathbf{p} \in M_c(Z) \mid \mathbf{p}$ satisfies the property $ç\}$. Define $I_c(P_i,M_c(Z,ç)) = \min\{I_c(P_i,\mathbf{p}) \mid \mathbf{p} \in M_c(Z,ç)\}$. If $M_c(Z,ç)=\emptyset$ then we let $I_c(P_i,M_c(Z,ç))=0$. Finaly, we say that $I_c(P_i,ç) = \max\{I_c(P_i,M_c(Z,ç)) \mid Z \subseteq X_i\}$ is the <u>information content of P_i according to c and ç</u>. In the case that every c-partition of P_i has the property ç we say that $I_c(P_i) = I_c(P_i,ç)$ is the <u>information content of P_i according to c</u>.

We note that $I_3(P_i)$ is defined as information content of P_i in |43|. So, the main extention of the original definition introduced here is based on taking a property ç into consideration. How can one use this ç ? One possibility is to find an convinient property $ç_U$ to a special model of VLSI circuits U in order to obtain some stronger lower bounds for the complexity measure AT^2 of U-circuits solving specific problems. This approach can lead to the design of optimal VLSI algorithms according to some special (suitable for the current technology) VLSI models. The second possibility is to consider whether there exists a restricting property ç such that $(I_c(P_i,ç))^2$ provides the lower bound on AT^2. Whether such a ç exists and can help in lower bound proving we let as the main open problem formulated here.

Now, we can formulate an algorithm for proving a lower bound on AT^2 for VLSI circuits of a type U described by the property $ç_U$.

" AT^2 algorithm "

Input: A problem instance P with the set of input variables X, the set of output variables Y, and a property $ç_U$.

Step1. Choose: a, a positive integer $c \geq 3$

b, a $Z \subseteq X$.

Step2. Let $\mathbf{p}_1, \mathbf{p}_2, \ldots, \mathbf{p}_s$ be all different c-partitions for P according to Z having the property $ç_U$. Find, for each i $\in \{1,2,3,\ldots,s\}$, $\mathbf{A}_i$ - the largest fooling set for $\mathbf{p}_i$.

Step3. Compute $d = \min\{|\mathbf{A}_i| \mid i=1,\ldots,s\}$.

Output: $$c^2 A(R)(T(R))^2 \geq (\log_2 d)^2$$

for every VLSI-circuit of the type U solving the problem instance P .

Now, we present a result showing that the B-circuits have a stronger relation to information transfer than the general VLSI-circuits.

Theorem 5.7 |43| Let $c \geq 3$ be a positive integer, and let $\mathbf{P} = \{P_i\}_{i=1}^{\infty}$ be a problem, where for each i the size of P_i is n_i and P_i depends on all n_i input variables. Let $\mathbf{R} = \{R_i\}_{i=1}^{\infty}$ be a sequence of B-circuits solving $\mathbf{P}$. Then

$$A_{\mathbf{R}}(n_i)(T_{\mathbf{R}}(n_i))^2 \geq n_i I_c(P_i)/4$$

for every positive integer i.

Proof. Let us consider the B-circuit R_i solving the problem instance P_i. Let the sides of R_i be m and s, where $m \geq s$. Since there is at most $2(m+s)$ input processors we obtain $T(R_i) \geq n_i/2(m+s) \geq n_i/4m$, i.e. $m \geq n_i/4T(R_i)$. On the other hand dividing the B-circuit R_i into two parts we obtain $sT(R_i) \geq I_c(P_i)$, i.e. $s \geq I_c(P_i)/T(R_i)$. So, we have $A(R_i) = sm \geq (I_c(P_i)/T(R_i))(n_i/4T(R_i)) = n_i I_c(P_i)/4(T(R_i))^2$ what implies $A(R_i)(T(R_i))^2 \geq n_i I_c(P_i)/4$.

Concluding this section we give an example showing how the property ç included in the definition of information content can help to obtain stronger lower bounds on AT^2 for a special VLSI model. Let FIX(1,1)-circuit is a B(1,1)-circuit such that if $z_1,\ldots,z_m$ is the order (from the left to the right or from up to down) of input processors leading on the input border then, for $1 \leq i < j \leq m$, each variable assigned to z_i has smaller index than any variable assigned to z_j.

Theorem 5.8 The simulation of a 1VLSI circuit solving a problem instance P of the size n by a FIX(1,1)-circuit can require $cn/(\log_2 n)^2$ increase of the complexity AT^2.

Proof: Let us consider the recognition of the language $L = \{ww \mid w \in \{0,1\}^*\}$, i.e. let us consider the sequence $\{f_i\}_{i=1}^{\infty}$ of Boolean functions, where f_i has i input variables and $f_i(x_1,x_2,\ldots,x_i)=1$ iff there is a $w \in \{0,1\}^*$ such that $x_1x_2\ldots x_i = ww$.

One can easy see that considering binary tree T as 4-graph with the input variables assigned to the i leaves in the order $x_1x_{(i/2)+1}x_2x_{(i/2)+2}\ldots x_{i/2}x_i$ from the left to the right leaf the 1VLSI circuit $\mathbf{R}$ can be constructed. Since the binary tree with n leaves can be laid out in the lattice as so-called H-tree |43| with area complexity $O(n)$ the designed 1VLSI circuit R has AT^2 in $O(n(\log_2 n)^2)$.

Now, let us show that each FIX(1,1)-circuit need AT^2 at least n^2/d for a constant d to solve f_n for n even. Without loss of the generality we can assume that the FIX(1,1) circuit solving f_n is a (n/4)FIX(1,1) circuit because f_n depends on all its input variables (what implies that a VLSI circuit having an input processor assigned to more than $n/4$ input variables has $T^2 \geq n^2/16$).

To prove our result it suffices to prove $I_4(f_n, \varsigma_{FIX}) \geq n/4$, where ς_{FIX} is the condition on partitions requiring, for any partition $\mathbf{p}=(Z,S_I,S_{II},Y_I,Y_{II})$ that $x_i \in S_I$ and $x_j \in S_{II}$ implies $i < j$. Let $X=\{x_1,\ldots,x_n\}$ be the set of input variables. We choose $Z=X$ and show that $I_4(f_n, M_4(Z,\varsigma_{FIX})) \geq n/4$. Let $\mathbf{p} \in M_4(Z,\varsigma_{FIX})$. Then $\mathbf{p}=(X,X_L,X_R,Y_L,Y_R)$, where $X_L=\{x_1,\ldots,x_m\}$ and $X_R=\{x_{m+1},\ldots,x_n\}$ for $n/4 \leq m \leq 3n/4$. In the case that $m \leq n/2$ we claim that the fooling set

$$\mathbf{A_p}=\{uvzy \mid v=y=1^{n/4},\ u=z \in \{0,1\}^{n/4}\},$$

and in the case $m > n/2$ we claim that the fooling set

$$\mathbf{A_p'}=\{uvzy \mid u=z=1^{n/4},\ v=y \in \{0,1\}^{n/4}\}.$$

We prove only that $\mathbf{A_p}$ is a fooling set since the proof for $\mathbf{A_p'}$ is very similar. We consider two possibilities:

(1) $Y_L = \{y\}$ and $Y_R = \emptyset$.

(2) $Y_L = \emptyset$ and $Y_R = \{y\}$.

Let $\mathbf{a}, \mathbf{b} \in \mathbf{A_p}$, $\mathbf{a} \neq \mathbf{b}$, and let $\mathbf{a} = u1^{n/4}u1^{n/4}$, $\mathbf{b} = v1^{n/4}v1^{n/4}$. Following this fact and $u \neq v$ we obtain $f_n(\mathbf{a}_L\mathbf{b}_R) = 0 \neq 1 = f_n(\mathbf{a})$. So, in the case (1) $f_n(\mathbf{a}_L\mathbf{b}_R)$ differs from $f_n(\mathbf{a})$ on the variable y in Y_L , in the case (2) $f_n(\mathbf{a}_L\mathbf{b}_R)$ differs from $f_n(\mathbf{a})$ on the variable y in Y_R .

Since $|\mathbf{A_p}| = 2^{n/4}$ we have for each $\mathbf{p} \in M_4(Z,\varsigma_{FIX})$ that $I_4(f_n,\mathbf{p}) \geq n/4$. This implies $I_4(f_n,\varsigma_{FIX}) \geq I_4(f_n,M_4(Z,\varsigma_{FIX})) \geq n/4$, i.e. $AT^2 \geq n^2/16$.

6. TOPOLOGY OF CIRCUITS AND INFORMATION TRANSFER

The framework for the study of information transfer in VLSI circuits was given in Section 5. We use this framework to obtain lower bound techniques for some special types of VLSI circuits determined by the VLSI topology. The lower bound arguments presented here have to motivate the reader to try to find optimal VLSI algorithms for some problems solved on the VLSI models considered here. We think that the results of this type can have both the theoretical significance and the practical applications.

One can consider VLSI circuits with VLSI graphs from some special classes of graphs in order to bring the regularity in VLSI design. It is well-known that the regularity of VLSI circuits has an essential influence on the reliability of produced chips, on the complexity of chip testing, and so on the charge of producing the VLSI chips. Because of the lack of the space we shall present only the relation between information content and two types of topological structures - linear arrays and balanced binary trees investigated intensively in several papers (see, for example, |7,8,11,21,22,36|).

Now, the question is what does the notion "topological regularity" mean ? A possible approach is the following one. Let us consider, for instance, the full (balanced) binary trees (FBT) as a regular structures. Now, we could define FBT-circuits as VLSI circuits whose 4-graph is an FBT. Clearly, this approach leads to the regularity of VLSI graphs. We say to this type of regularity the "total regularity" that is not often used this tyme because it requires the regularity of the VLSI circuit design in the smallest details. So, we define the regularity according to the graph topology in a more general way that corresponds to the fact that the VLSI circuit designers are working with processors and wires computing over a finite alphabet (not only in the two-valued logic).

Definition 6.1 Let k be a positive integer, and let $\mathbf{G}$ be a class (set) of undirected graphs. By $EM_k(\mathbf{G})$ we denote the set of k-regular graphs according to $\mathbf{G}$ that involves each directed 4-graph $G'=(V',E')$ that can be obtained from a graph $G=(V,E)\in\mathbf{G}$ by replacing every vertex $v\in V$ by a directed graph G_v having at most k vertices, and by replacing every edge $(u,v)\in E$ by at most k directed edges, each leading from a $z_1\in G_u$ (G_v) to a $z_2\in G_v$ (G_u). The positive number k is called the degree of nonregularity .

Definition 6.2 Let $\mathbf{G}$ denote a class of undirected graphs. We denote by $\mathbf{G}_k$-circuit the VLSI circuits having their VLSI-graphs in $EM_k(\mathbf{G})$. The class of undirected, balanced binary trees will be denoted by BT, the class of linear (one-dimensional) arrays (an array can be viewed as a tree having exactly two leaves) will be denoted by 1A.

In Definitions 6.1 and 6.2 we have defined the base for topological regularity that corresponds to the designer's approach assuming that the processors in the vertices of VLSI graphs have a constant memory and compute over a finite alphabet. It follows from the fact that each processor working over a finite alphabet can be understood as a VLSI graph with constant number of processors computing over the alphabet $\{0,1\}$.

Now, we relate the information content of a problem to the time complexity of BT_k-circuits and $1A_k$-circuits. Why can the information content provide direct lower bounds on time ? It follows from the approach based on dividing the VLSI circuit into two parts by removing some suitable wires (edges). The choise of the wires for removing is independent on the embeding of the graph into lattice. This was not the case in the previous section, where all removed wires were those ones which crossed the line dividing the lattice into two parts.

First, let us study $1A_k$-circuits known as two-way one-dimensional systolic arrays from the literature.

Theorem 6.3 Let k be a positive integer. Let P be a problem instance depending on all its input variables with the information content $I_k(P)$. Then

$$T \geq I_k(P)/2k$$

for any $1A_k$-circuit solving P .

Proof. Let M be a $1A_k$-circuit solving P . Let X be the set of input variables of P , and let $Z \subseteq X$ such that $I_k(P)=I_k(P,Z)=I_k(P,M_k(Z,ç))$, where ç is a property of all partitions. In the case that M is not a $(|Z|/k)$VLSI circuit there is a processor of M that has assigned at least $|Z|/k + 1$ input variables. This implies $T(M) \geq |Z|/k \geq I_k(P)/k$.

So, we can assume that M is a $(|Z|/k)$VLSI circuit. Now, it is sufficient to find $2k$ edges in the VLSI graph of M dividing the VLSI graph into two parts in such a way that the number a (b) of input variables assigned to the left (right) part (see Fig.3) fulfils $|Z|/2 - |Z|/k \leq a\ (b) \leq |Z|/2 + |Z|/k$.

Figure 3.:

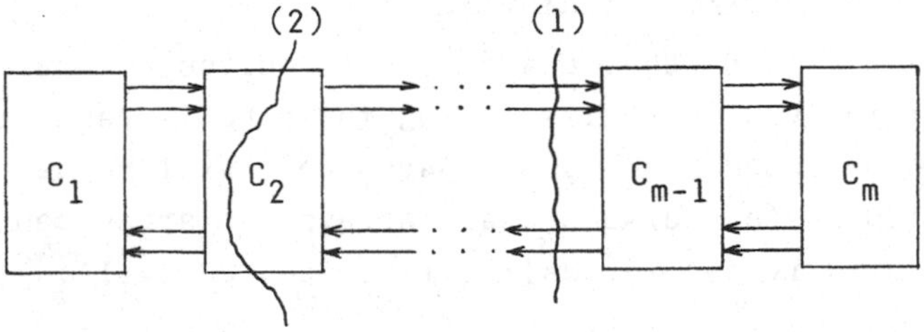

Clearly, M can be understood as the circuit at Fig.3 consisting of m components $C_1, C_2, \ldots, C_m$, for a positive integer m , where there are at most k edges between components C_i and C_{i+j} for $j < 2$, and any component involves at most k processors connected by at most $2k$ edges. We can find the partitioning of M in the following way. Let C_i be the component with the smallest i such that $d \geq |Z|/2 - |Z|/k$ input variables from Z are assigned to the components $C_1, C_2, \ldots, C_i$. If $d \leq |Z|/2 + |Z|/k$ then removing the edges between C_i and C_{i+1} (see the line of the type (1) at Fig.3) we obtain the required partition. If $d > |Z|/2 + |Z|/k$ then we have to divide the component

C_i into two components C_i^1 and C_i^2 (see the line of the type (2) at Fig.3). Clearly, removing at most $2k$ edges we can divide M into two parts (one consisting from the components $C_1, C_2, \ldots, C_{i-1}, C_i^1$ and the other one from the components $C_i^2, C_{i+1}, C_{i+2}, \ldots, C_m$) such that at least $|Z|/2 - |Z|/k$ input variables are assigned to each side.

We have proved that each two-way one-dimensional systolic array solving a problem instance P has the time complexity at least $I_3(P)/2k$, where k is the degree of nonregularity. It means that we can speed up the computation according to $I_3(P)$ only by using a higher degree of nonregularity of two-way one-dimensional systolic arrays. Now, we shall present similar results for a more general VLSI model based in the topology of binary trees.

Theorem 6.4 Let k be a positive integer. Let P be a problem instance depending on all its n input variables with the information content $I_k(P)$. Then

$$T(M) \geq I_k(P)/k^2 \log_2 2m$$

for any BT_k-circuit M with $2m-1$ vertices solving P .

Proof. Let k be a positive integer. Let P be a problem instance depending on all its n input variables with the information content $I_k(P)$. Let M be a BT_k-circuit solving P . Let X be the set of input variables of P , and let $Z \subseteq X$ such that $I_k(P) = I_k(P, M_k(Z, ç))$, where ç is the property of all partitions. In the case that M is not a $(|Z|/k^2)$VLSI circuit there is a processor of M that has assigned at least $|Z|/k^2 + 1$ input variables. This implies $T(M) \geq |Z|/K^2 \geq I_k(P)/k^2$.

So, we can assume that M is a $(|Z|/k^2)$VLSI circuit which implies that at most n/k input variables are assigned to any component of k processors of M corresponding to a vertex of the binary tree. Now, it is sufficient to find $\log_2 2m$ edges ($k\log_2 2m$ wires) in the full binary tree (in M) dividing the tree (M) into two parts in such a way that the number a of input variables from Z assigned to the components in the "left" part fulfils $|Z|/2 - |Z|/k \leq a \leq |Z|/2 + |Z|/k$.

An algorithm that find this division of M can work on the full binary tree F (that is laid in the plane in the usual way as a planar graph) as follows. It starts taking the left-most leaf in the left part, and taking all other vertices of F in the right part. Let $a <$ $|Z|/2 - |Z|/k$, and let all i vertices in the left part have all their sons in the left part after i step of the algorithm. The (i+1)-th step of the algorithm consists in taking one vertex v from the right part and giving it in the left part. To choose v we consider the following criteria with the significance in the presented order.

(1) All sons (if v is a non-leaf) of v are in the left part.

(2) If no non-leaf vertex v with the property (1) exists take the left-most leaf of F .

We note that the algorithm gives an order of vertices of F (see Fig.4, where the vertices of the full binary tree with 8 leaves are orderd). Clearly, if we choose the vertex v fulfilling (1) the number

Figure 4.:

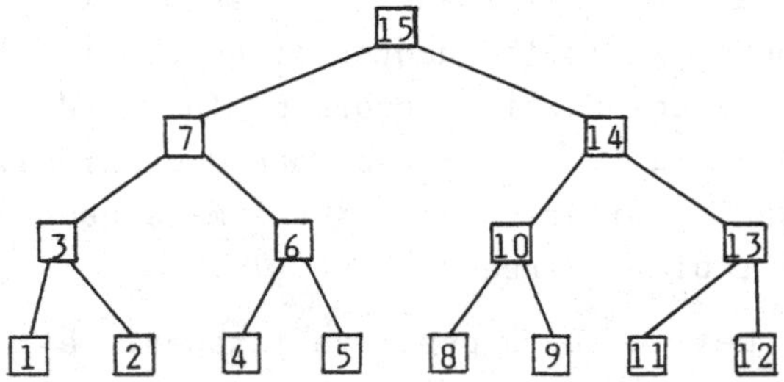

of edges between the left part and the right part of F is decreased by 1 (there are the cases in which the internal vertices 3,6,7,10,13,14,15 were chosen from the tree at Fig.4). In the case in which we choose a leaf according to (2) the number of edges between the left part and the right one is increased by 1. One can simple seen that, for any positive integer i , there are only the two following possibilities concerning the edges between the two parts:

(a) There is at most one edge in each level of F that connects the two parts (this situation is after choosing the vertices 1,3,4,7,8, 10,11 from the tree at Fig.4).

(b) There is a level j involving two edges connecting the left part with the right one, no edge from the levels 1,2,...,j-1 connects these two parts, and at most one edge from levels $j+1,j+2,\dots,\log_2 m$ connects these two parts.

Since the number of levels of the full binary tree F with 2m-1 vertices is exactly $\log_2 m$ we have shown that, for any $i = 1,2,\dots,2m-1$, there are at most $\log_2 m + 1 = \log_2 2m$ edges between two parts of F obtained by the lagorithm after i steps.

Obviously, we can stop the algorithm after the first step in which $a \le |Z|/2 - |Z|/k$. Since M is an $(|Z|/k^2)$VLSI circuit $a \le |Z|/2 + |Z|/k$ and we have obtained the required division of M according to the partition of input variables from Z .

The assertion of Theorem 6.4 claims that if we want to speed up a VLSI computation on full binary trees we need to use very large trees. For example it implies that a problem with the information transfer

$I_k(n) = \Omega(n)$ requires a full binary tree with

$$\Omega(2^{n/\log_2 n})$$

verticse to be solved in logarithmic time. One can ask whether it is possible to construct such a fast circuit with so large number of processors. Now, we claim that it is impossible.

Theorem 6.5 Let $f: N \rightarrow N$ be an increasing function. Let $k \geq 3$ be a positive integer and let $P = \{P_i\}_{i=1}$ be a problem. Let, for each $i \in N$, $|P_i| = i$ and each output variable of P_i depends on all i input variables. Then there is no sequence $R = \{R_i\}_{i=1}^{\infty}$ of FBT_k-circuits solving P with

$$T_R(n) \leq (I_k(P_n))^{1/2}/f(n)$$

for infinitely many n.

Corollary 6.6 Let $P = \{P_i\}_{i=1}$ be a problem with the information content $I_k(P_i) \geq i^a$ for a constant $0 < a < 1$. Then there is no sequence R of FBT_k-circuits solving P in polylogarithmic time.

The proof of Theorem 2.5 Let, for any positive integer i, R_i be an FBT_k-circuit solving P_i with $T(R_i) \leq (I_k(P_i))^{1/2}/f(n)$. Let R_i be minimal FBT_k-circuit according to the number of processors with the above formulated properties. Using Theorem 6.4 we have we have that $T(R_i) \geq I_k(P_i)/k^2\log_2 2m$, where m is the number of leaf-components of R_i. It implies that $k^2\log_2 2m \geq f(n)(I_k(P_i))^{1/2}$, i.e.

$$2m \geq 2^{f(i)(I_k(P_i))^{1/2}/k^2}$$

Let x_r, x_s be two input variables assigned to the processors v_r and v_s respectively. The distance between the processors v_r and v_s can be at most $T(R_i) \leq (I_k(P_i))^{1/2}/f(i)$ because in the opposite case there exists no output variable y depending on both input variables x_r and x_s. So, there exists a processor p in R_i such that all input and output processors has the distance from p at most $2(I_k(P_i))^{1/2}/f(n)$, i.e. all processors whose output values have an influence on the value of an output variable have their distance from p at most $3(I_k(P_i))^{1/2}/f(i)$. Let us call these processors the active processors.

Since there is the processor p with the distance at most $3(I_k(P_i))^{1/2}/f(i)$ to any active processor there is a binary subtree T_1 of the high at most $6(I_k(P_i))^{1/2}/f(i)$ involving all active processors.

It can be simply seen that there is an n_0 such that for all $i \geq n_0$:

$$2m \geq 2^{f(i)(I_k(P_i))^{1/2}/k^2} \geq 8 \cdot 2^{6(I_k(P_i))^{1/2}/f(i)}$$

which implies that for all $i \geq n_0$ the FBT_k-circuit R_i is not minimal according to the number of processors (obviously, all non-active processors of R_i can be deleted without changing the problem solved by R_i). This is a contradiction to our assumption completeng the proof .

Following the above stated assertions we formulate some motivations for futher research.

Motivation 6.7 Is the result of Theorem 2.5 the best possible for full binary trees ? It means that the question is whether there is a problem $P = \{P_i\}_{i=1}^{\infty}$ such that we can construct a sequence $R = \{R_i\}_{i=1}^{\infty}$ of FBT_k-circuits solving P with $T_R(n) \leq (I_k(P_n))^{1/2}$ or such a problem does not exist. In the case that such a problem does not exist try to improve the assertion of Theorem 6.5 .

Motivation 6.8 Consider a full binary tree or one-dimensional systolic array with fixed number of vertices m as a regular VLSI models. Try to find optimal VLSI algorithms solving some specific problems on these regular VLSI models according to the time complexity measure.

Now, we shall present (without proofs according to bounded area complexity of this paper) a lower bound technique for a more specific model - the binary tree automata as introduced in |7,8| (The binary tree automata, BTAs, have the input variables assigned to the leaves of BTAs, the information is flowing only in the direction from the leaves to the root, and they are working in time $\log_2 n$ on problem instances of the size n).

Lemma 6.9 Let k be a positive integer. Let L be a language recognized by a BTA automaton. Then there is a constant d such that

$$I_k(h_n^L, \varsigma_{FIX}) \leq d\log_2 n .$$

Lemma 6.10 Let k be a positive integer. Let L be a language recognized by a BTA automaton. Then there exists a constant d such that

$$I_k(h_n^L, \varsigma_{FIX}) \leq d$$

for all $n=2^m$, $m \in N$.

Clearly, the above presented results claim that it is not reasonable to consider the tree structure for computing problems with high information content.

7. COMMUNICATION COMPLEXITY

The abstraction of the concept of information transfer led to the definition of the notion "communication complexity" for language recognition in |30|. Let us give an informal definition of this complexity measure.

Suppose that a language $L \subseteq (\{0,1\}^2)^*$ must be recognized by two distant computers. Each computer receives half of the input bits, and the computation proceeds using some protocols for communication between the two computers. The minimum number of bits that has to be exchanged in order to successfully recognize $L \cap \{0,1\}^n$, minimized over all partitions of the input bits into two equal-sided parts, and considered as a function of n, is called the communication complexity of L .

This complexity measure was studied in several papers |3,9, 12-16,18,24,25,30|. In the original paper of Papadimitriou and Sipser |30| it was proved that one communication bit helps to recognize more languages, most languages required maximal communication complexity, the nondeterministic communication complexity was defined and an exponential gap between determinism and nondeterminism in communication complexity was shown. On the other hand Ďuriš, Galil and Schnitger |9| has proved that one bit can help more than nondeterminism.

Closure properties of the families of languages determined by communication complexity were investigated in |3,12|. In |12| there are found two languages L_1 and L_2 such that L_1 and L_2 have constant communication complexity and the languages $L_1 \cup L_2$ and $L_1 \cap L_2$ have linear communication complexity. These results were extended to the nondeterministic case in |3|, where it was proved that allmost all languages L have the property that both L and L^c require maximal nondeterministic communication complexity too.

Using communication complexity Gubáš and Waczulík |13| proved that there are two languages W_1 and W_2 that can be recognized in $O(n(\log_2 n)^3)$ AT^2 complexity, but the recognition of $W_1 \cup W_2$ require $n^2/(\log_2 n)^3$ AT^2 complexity.

Several special types of communication complexity were investigated in |9,14,16,18,30| in order to go deeper in the understanding of the nature of communication complexity.

A new approach in information transfer |2| motivated for a new, generalized definition of communication complexity in |18|, where the basic properties of generalized communication complexity are proved, the differences between the original communication complexity and the generalized communication complexity are shown, the NP-completness of the problem of determination whether a given problem instance has non-zero communication complexity was presented, and several motivations for futher research are formulated. The unclosure properties of generalized communication comlexity follows from |13|. Several motivations for futher research in communication complexity theory are formulated in |20-23| too.

8. INFORMATION TRANSFER AND LOWER BOUNDS FOR OTHER COMPLEXITY MEASURES

We shall outline in this section how the idea based on information content (or communication complexity) was used to obtain lower bounds for distinct computing models.

8.1 Area and space complexity of Boolean circuits

The problem of determining lower bounds on area and space needed for computing some special problems on the well-known computing models - Boolean circuits was investigated in |39,40|, where the lower bound $\Omega(n^{3/2})$ for a specific Boolean function was established. Using a special type of communication complexity the strongest-known lower bounds $\Omega(n^2)$ and $\Omega(n^{3/2})$ resp. was obtained for the area and space complexity respectively in |19|.

8.2 Linear lower bounds for CA-circuits

The CA-circuits introduced in |17| are a generalization of unbounded fan-in Boolean circuits. Defining the communication complexity of CA-circuits the method for obtaining linear lower bounds on the number of gates was developed in |17|.

8.3 Lower bounds on branching programs

The branching programs were introduced in |29,35| as a tool for obtaining lower bounds on the space complexity of sequential algorithms. A special type of communication complexity was used to obtain new lower bounds for branching programs |34|. In some sence this special communication complexity is related to the width of branching programs.

8.4 Information flow among distinct processes in distributed computing

The communication complexity model can be used to study the requirements on the information flow among distinct processes in distributed computing |1,24|. The question whether the computation facilities of special communication computers in a computer network with a special topology can decrease the amount of submitted data is investigated .

ACKNOWLEDGEMENT

I would very like to thank **Tánička** for her patience and help during the preparation of the final version of this paper.

REFERENCES

1. **Abelson,H.**: Lower bounds on information transfer in distributed computations. Proc. 19th Annual IEEE FOCS, IEEE 1978, pp. 151-158.

2. **Aho,A.V. - Ullman,J.D. - Yanakakis,M.**: On notions of information transfer in VLSI circuits. Proc. 15th ACM STOC, ACM 1983, pp. 133-139.

3. **Bačík,M.**: Closure properties of communication complexity. ŠVOČ 1987, 1, section Theoretical Cybernetics and Mathematical Informatics, Comenius University, Bratislava 1987, 12p. (in Slovak).

4. **Baudet,G.M.**: On the area required by VLSI circuits. In: Kung, Sproul, and Steele 1981, pp. 100-107.

5. **Brent,R.P. - Goldschlager,L.M.**: Some area time tradeoffs for VLSI. SIAM J. Comput. 11, No.4 (1982), pp. 737-747.

6. **Brent,R.P. - Kung,H.T.**: The chip complexity of binary arithmetic. Proc. 12th Annual ACM STOC, ACM 1980, pp. 190-200.

7. **Culik,K.II. - Gruska,J. - Salomaa,A.**: Systolic automata for VLSI on balanced trees. Acta Informat. 18 (1983), 335-344.

8. **Culik,K.II. - Gruska,J. - Salomaa,A.**: On a family of L languages resulting from systolic tree automata. Theor. Comp. Sci. 23 (1983), 231-242.

9. **Ďuriš,P. - Galil,Z. - Schnitger,G.**: Lower bounds on communication complexity. Proc. 15th Annual ACM STOC, ACM 1984, pp. 81-91.

10. **Ďuriš,P. - Sýkora,O. - Vrťo,I. - Thompson,C.D.**: Tight chip lower bounds for discrete Fourier and Walsh-Hadamard transformations. Infor. Proces. Let. 21 (1985), 245-247.

11. **Gruska,J.**: Systolic automata - power, characterizations, nonhomogenity. Proc. 11th MFCS´84, Lect. Notes in Computer Science 176, Springer-Verlag, Berlin Heidelberg-New York 1984, pp. 32-49.

12. **Gubáš,X. - Waczulík,J.**: Closure properties of the family of languages defined ba communication complexity. ŠVOČ 1986, 1, section Theoretical Cybernetics and Mathematical Informatics, Comenius University, Bratislava 1986, 26p. (in Slovak).

13. **Gubáš,X. - Waczulík,J.**: Closure properties of the complexity measures A and AT^2. ŠVOČ 1987, 1, section VLSI and Computer Graphics. Comenius University, Bratislava 1987, 25p. (in Slovak).

14. **Hromkovič,J.**: Communication complexity. Proc. 11th ICALP, Lect. Notes in Computer Science 172, Springer-Verlag, Berlin-Heidelberg-New York 1984, pp. 235-246.

15. **Hromkovič, J.**: Relation between Chomsky hierarchy and communication complexity hierarchy. Acta Math. Univ. Com. 47-48 (1986).

16. **Hromkovič,J.**: Normed protocol and communication complexity. Computers AI 3, No.5 (1984), 415-422.

17. **Hromkovič,J.**: Linear lower bounds on unbounded fan-in Boolean circuits. Infor. Proces. Let. 21 (1985), 71-74.

18. **Hromkovič,J.**: A new approach to defining the communication complexity for VLSI. Proc. 12th MFCS´86, Lect. Notes in Computer Science 233, Springer-Verlag, Berlin-Heidelberg-New York 1986, pp. 431-439.

19. **Hromkovič,J. - Ložkin,C.A. - Rybko,A.N. - Sapoženko,A.A. - Škalikova, N.A.**: An approach to obtaining lower bounds on space of Boolean circuits. Banach Centre publ., to appear (In Russian).

20. **Hromkovič,J.**: Some complexity aspects of VLSI computations, Part 1.: A framework for the study of information transfer in VLSI circuits. Submitted to Computers AI.

21. **Hromkovič,J.**: Some complexity aspects of VLSI computations. Part 2.: Topology of circuits and information transfer. Submitted to Computers AI.

23. **Hromkovič,J.**: Some complexity aspects of VLSI computations. Part 5.: Nondeterministic and probabilistic VLSI circuits. Submitted to Computer AI.

24. **Hromkovič,J. - Pardubská,A.**: Some complexity aspects of VLSI computations. Part 3.: On the power of input bit permutation in tree and trellis automata. Submitted to Computers AI.

24. **Ja´Ja,J. - Prasanna Kumar,V.K. - Simon,J.**: Information transfer under different sets of protocols. SIAM J. Comput. 13, No.4 (1984), 840-849.

25. **Kurcabová,V.**: Communication complexity. Master thesis, Dept. of Theor. Cybernetics, Comenius University, Bratislava 1985 (in Slovak).

26. **Leiserson,C.E.**: Area efficient graph algorithms (for VLSI). Proc. 21st Annual IEEE FOCS, IEEE 1980, pp. 270-281.

27. **Leiserson,C.E.**: Area efficient VLSI computations. MIT Press, Cambridge 1983, Mass.

28. **Lipton,R.J. - Sedgewick,R.**: Lower bounds for VLSI. Proc. 13th Annual ACM STOC, ACM 1981, pp. 300-307.

29. **Masek,W.**: A fast algorithm for string editing problem and decision graph complexity. M.Sc. thesis, MIT, May 1976.

30. **Papadimitriou,C.H. - Sipser,M.**: Communication complexity. J.Comp. Syst. Sci. 28 (1984), 260-269.

31. **Preparata,F.P.**: A mesh-connected area-time optimal VLSI integer multiplier. In: Kung, Sproull, and Steele 1981, pp. 311-316.

32. **Preparata,F.P. - Vuilemin,J.E.**: Area-time optimal VLSI networks for multiplying matrices. Infor. Proces. Let. 11, No.2 (1980), 77-80.

33. **Preparata,F.P. - Vuilemin,J.E.**: Area-time optimal VLSI networks for computing integer multiplication and discrete Fourier transformation. Proc. 8th ICALP´81, Lect. Notes in Computer Science 115, Springer-Verlag, Berlin-Heidelberg-New York 1981, pp. 29-40.

34. **Pudlák,P.**: personal communication.

35. **Pudlák,P. - Žák,S.**: Space complexity of computations. Unpublished manuscript, 1982.

36. **Salomaa,A.**: Systolic tree and trellis automata. Proc. Collq. ACLCS, Gyor 1984.

37. **Savage,J.E.**: Planar circuit complexity and the performance of VLSI algorithms. In: Kung, Sproul, and Steele, 1981, pp. 61-67.

38. **Savage,J.E.**: Area-time tradeoffs for mutrix multiplication and related problems in VLSI models. J. Comp. Syst. Sci. 20, No.3, pp. 230-242.

39. **Škalikova,N.A.**: On the area complexity of Boolean circuits computing some specific functions. Sbornik rabot po matematičeskoj kibernetike I (1976), Comp. Centre of the Academy of Sciences of USSR,pp. 102-115 (in Russian).

40. **Škalikova,N.A.**: On the relation between area and space complexity of Boolean circuits. Metody diskretnogo analiza v ocenkach zložnosti upravľajuščich sistem 38, Novosibirsk 1982, pp. 87-107 (in Russian).

41. **Thompson,C.D.**: Area-time complexity for VLSI. Proc. 11th Annual ACM STOC, ACM 1979, pp. 81-88.

42. **Thompson,C.D.**: A Complexity Theory for VLSI. Doctoral dissertation,

CMU-CS-80-140, Computer Sci. Dept., Carnegie - Mellon University, Pittsburg, August 1980, 131p.

43. **Ullman,A.C.**: Computational Aspects of VLSI. Computer SCience Press 1984, 495p.

44. **Yao,A.C.**: Some complexity questions related to distributed computing. Proc. 11th Annual ACM STOC, ACM 1979, pp. 209-213.

35. **Yao,A.C.**: The entropic limitations of VLSI computations. Proc. 13th Annual ACM STOC, ACM 1981, pp. 308-311.

THE EQUIVALENCE OF MAPPINGS ON LANGUAGES

Juhani Karhumäki
Department of Mathematics
University of Turku
20500 Turku, Finland

Abstract. We define the notion of the equivalence of mappings on languages in three different ways and call them universal equivalence, existential equivalence and equivalence with multiplicities. We survey recent results on this topic, as well as state some open problems.

1. Introduction

Since the beginning of the automata theory one of the most natural problems of the field has been the equivalence problem for automata or other devices of a certain type, that is to say, the problem of finding an algorithm or proving the nonexistence of such to decide whether two given automata behave in the same way, or in other words, are equivalent. Our intention here is to point out that the research in this problem area is still now - 30 years later - quite active and that there are many attractive unanswered problems left.

We formulate our basic problem as follows. Let $\mathcal{L}$ be a family of languages over a finite alphabet Σ and θ a family of (not necessarily single-valued) partial mappings or devices defining such from the free monoid Σ^* into another free monoid. Then we want to decide whether, for a given L from $\mathcal{L}$ and two mappings from θ, these mappings are "equivalent" on L. This problem in connection with morphisms, i.e., the "morphic equivalence for languages", was introduced by Culik and Salomaa in [CS], which was a starting point for quite an active research.

Clearly, the above formulation includes the problem of deciding the equivalence of two automata with outputs, i.e., the equivalence problem for finite transducers. Other typical cases we shall be dealing with are the cases when $\mathcal{L}$ is the family of regular languages and θ is either a morphic mapping, i.e., a composition of morphisms and inverse morphisms, or a finite substitution. In particular, we shall be looking for borderlines between the decidable and undecidable equivalence problems in these cases.

If the partial mappings σ and τ are many-valued, in other words nondeterministic, then there are (at least) three different possibilities to define the notion of the equivalence of σ and τ on L. In each case the equivalence is word-by-word equivalence, which means that the mappings must behave in a similar way on each of the words of L. The most natural definition of the equivalence is the ordinary one which we refer to as the universal equivalence: σ and τ are universally equivalent on a word x if $\sigma(x)$ and $\tau(x)$ coincide as sets. They are existentially equivalent on x if either $\sigma(x)$ and $\tau(x)$ have a nonempty intersection or both are empty, and they are equivalent with multiplicities if $\sigma(x)$ and $\tau(x)$ are the same as multisets.

The rest of this paper is organized as follows.

After introducing the problems in details in Section 2 we recall in Section 3 the main decidability and undecidability results concerning the (universal) equivalence problem for transducers. We consider both one-way and two-way finite transducers, but do not deal with more general devices. Some of the results are rather new and are obtained by using techniques which allow to test the equivalence not only on the domains of the transducers but also on a given HDTOL language.

In Section 4 we consider the universal equivalence problem for different kinds of morphic and related mappings on regular languages. We are able to detect a sharp borderline between the decidability and the undecidability.

Finally, in Section 5 we discuss two other types of equivalences, although we have only a few results in this direction. We conclude this paper by giving a couple of open problems which, we believe, are quite interesting and important.

As a survey this paper does not contain any essentially new results. Neither are the proofs given, only a few outlines or simple constructions are shown. However, the references to complete works are always mentioned.

2. Preliminaries and the problems

We assume that the reader is familiar with the basics of formal language theory, cf. [H] or [Be]. Consequently, we recall here only very few definitions.

According to [Be] we denote a finite one-way transducer by a sixtuple $T = \langle\Sigma,\Delta,Q,q_0,F,E\rangle$, where Σ and Δ are the input and output alphabets respectively, Q is the set of states, q_0 is the initial state, F is the set of final states and $E \subseteq Q\times\Sigma^*\times\Delta^*\times Q$ is the set of transitions. The relation realized by T is denoted by $|T|$ and it can be viewed as a partial many-valued mapping from Σ^* into Δ^*. Forgetting the output structure of T we obtain the underlying finite (generalized) automaton of T.

Clearly, a finite transducer may produce an infinite number of outputs for a given input. However, in many cases we want to consider only the following restricted classes of transducers: (i) T is k-valued, for some given $k \geq 1$, if for each input word there exists at most k different output words, (ii) T is k-ambiguous, for some given $k \geq 1$, if for each input word there exists at most k different accepting computations, and (iii) T is deterministic if $E \subseteq Q \times \Sigma \times \Delta^* \times Q$ and for each $q \in Q$ and $a \in \Sigma$ the cardinality of the set $(\{q\} \times \{a\} \times \Delta^* \times Q) \cap E$ is at most one. Further a transducer is finite-valued (resp. finite-ambiguous) if it is k-valued (resp. k-ambiguous) for some $k \geq 1$. Observe also that our deterministic transducers are often called deterministic gsm's or deterministic sequential transducers. (Indeed, T is a gsm if $E \subseteq Q \times \Sigma \times \Delta^* \times Q$).

All the above restrictions can be defined in a natural way in connection with two-way finite transducers as well, cf. [EY].

Next we fix our notation for some families of partial mappings. We assume that the domain and range alphabets are fixed, say Σ and Δ. We denote by $\mathcal{H}$ and $\mathcal{S}$ the families of morphisms and finite substitutions, respectively. Clearly, each partial many-valued mapping σ considered as a relation has the inverse and thus defines the unique such mapping, the inverse of σ which is denoted by σ^{-1}. Similarly, any composition of such mappings defines the unique such mapping. Consequently, if θ_1 and θ_2 are families of partial many-valued mappings so are θ_1^{-1} and $\theta_1 \circ \theta_2$ (where we first apply mappings from θ_2). In particular, $\mathcal{H}^{-1}$ denotes inverse morphisms and $\mathcal{H}^{-1} \circ \mathcal{H}$ mappings of the form a morphism followed by an inverse morphism. Finally, we denote by $1\mathcal{T}$ (resp. $2\mathcal{T}$) the families of mappings defined by one-way (resp. two-way) finite transducers and we put in front of these abbreviations $\mathcal{D}$, $k\mathcal{V}$, $k\mathcal{A}$, $\mathcal{FV}$ and $\mathcal{FA}$ to denote deterministic, k-valued, k-ambiguous, finite-valued or finite-ambiguous restrictions, respectively.

We denote by Reg and $\mathcal{CF}$ the families of regular and context-free languages (over Σ). Further by $\mathcal{HDTOL}$ we mean the family of HDTOL languages, cf. [RS], defined as follows. Let w be a word over an alphabet Γ and $h_1, \ldots, h_k$, for some $k \geq 1$, morphisms from Γ^* into itself and f another morphism from Γ^* into Σ^*. We define the language

$$L = \bigcup_{i=0}^{\infty} f(L_i) ,$$

where

$$L_0 = \{w\}$$

$$L_{i+1} = h_1(L_i) \cup \ldots \cup h_k(L_i) \quad \text{for } i \geq 0 ,$$

and call languages L thus obtained HDTOL languages. It is straightforward to see that Reg $\subseteq$ *HDTOL*, and can be shown that the families *CF* and *HDTOL* are incomparable, cf. [NRSS].

Now, we formulate our problems. As earlier let Σ and Δ be two fixed finite alphabets. Further let L be a family of languages over Σ and θ a family of partial many-valued mappings from Σ^* into Δ^*. We say that mappings σ and τ universally (resp. existentially or with multiplicities) agree or are equivalent on a word $x \in \Sigma^*$ if

$$\sigma(x) = \tau(x) \quad \text{as ordinary sets} \tag{1}$$

$$(\text{resp. } \sigma(x) \cap \tau(x) \neq \phi \quad \text{whenever} \quad \sigma(x) \cup \tau(x) \neq \phi) \tag{2}$$

$$(\text{resp. } \sigma(x) = \tau(x) \quad \text{as multisets}) \tag{3}$$

Further we say that σ and τ agree (universally, existentially or with multiplicities) on a language $L \subseteq \Sigma^*$ if they do so on each of its words. We denote by

$$EP_{\forall}\ (\theta, L)$$

$$(\text{resp. } EP_{\exists}\ (\theta, L)\ )$$

$$(\text{resp. } EP_{M}\ (\theta, L)\ )$$

the problem of deciding whether two given mappings from θ are universally (resp. existentially or with multiplicities) equivalent on a given language from L. We refer these problems to as universal, existential and multiplicity θ-equivalence problems for L.

It follows immediately that for single-valued partial mappings the above three types of equivalences coincide. Observe also that in the definition of the equivalence with multiplicities the mappings σ and τ actually must be considered as mappings into the set of formal power series over nonnegative integers (augmented with ∞), i.e., into $\mathbb{N}^{(\infty)}\langle\langle\Delta^*\rangle\rangle$ in terms of [SS]. However, we shall be dealing with this notion only in connection with mappings defined by finite transducers, and since in this case the notion of "equality as multisets" meaning that the transducers must produce, for each input word, each output word equally many times is so intuitive and clear, we prefer not to go into a more formalized presentation.

3. The equivalence problem for transducers

In this section we consider the equivalence problem for different types of finite transducers. Here the equivalence means the universal equivalence so that in our earlier formulation the problem is $EP_{\forall}(\theta,\Sigma^*)$, where θ is (the family of mappings defined by) the corresponding family of transducers. Since the domains of all the transducers defined in the previous section are regular it follows that $EP_{\forall}(\theta,\Sigma^*)$ is equivalent to $EP_{\forall}(\theta,\mathrm{Reg})$ for all these families of transducers.

Our aim here is to point out a borderline between decidable and undecidable equivalence problems for finite transducers. To start with we first recall that the problem for all one-way finite transducers is undecidable as shown in [FR] and at the same time even in a slightly stronger form in [Gr]:

Theorem 1. The equivalence problem for λ-free nondeterministic gsm's (sequential transducers) is undecidable.

A striking generalization of this result was proved by Ibarra in [I1]:

Theorem 2. The equivalence problem for λ-free nondeterministic gsm's (sequential transducers) with unary output alphabet is undecidable.

As regards deterministic transducers it seems to us that the decidability of the equivalence problem for these has been known for a long time, a special case is covered already in [Mo], cf. also [Bi] and [JL], but the original proof can be found nowhere. In other words, the result seems to be considered as folklore. We present here a proof which is (after knowing some elementary automata theory) very simple and which also allows some generalizations.

Theorem 3. The equivalence problem for deterministic finite transducers is decidable.

Proof. Let $M_i = \langle\Sigma,\Delta,Q_i,q_i,F_i,E_i\rangle$, for $i = 1,2$, be two deterministic finite transducers. We define an infinite state automaton $A_\infty = \langle Q,q,F,\sigma\rangle$ as follows:

$$Q = Q_1 \times Q_2 \times \Delta^{(*)}$$

$$q = (q_1,q_2,\lambda)$$

$$F = \{(q,q',\lambda) \mid q \in F_1, q' \in F_2\}$$

$$\sigma((p_1,p_2,o),a) = (q_1,q_2,u_1^{-1}ou_2) \quad \text{if}$$

$$(p_i,a,u_i,q_i) \in E_i \quad \text{for} \quad i = 1,2 \; .$$

Here $\Delta^{(*)}$ denotes the free group generated by Δ. For each q in Q let us denote by length(q) the length of the (reduced) word in the third component of q. Now, for each $k \geq 1$, let A_k be the subautomaton of A_∞ obtained from it by removing all the states q (and corresponding transitions) for which length(q) > k.

Clearly, A_∞ is deterministic and

$$L(A_\infty) \subseteq \mathrm{dom}(T_1) \cap \mathrm{dom}(T_2) \tag{4}$$

It also follows from the construction that T_1 and T_2 are equivalent if and only if

$$L(A_\infty) = \mathrm{dom}(T_1) = \mathrm{dom}(T_2) \tag{5}$$

But now $\mathrm{dom}(T_1)$ and $\mathrm{dom}(T_2)$ are regular and hence (5) holds (remember (4)) if and only if

$$\exists k \geq 0 \text{ such that } L(A_k) = \mathrm{dom}(T_1) = \mathrm{dom}(T_2) \tag{6}$$

This last equivalence is a consequence of the following three facts:
(i) The minimal automaton for deterministic infinite state automaton is finite if and only if it accepts a regular language, cf. [E];
(ii) In each single step of a computation of A_∞ the length of a state can not decrease by more than a fixed constant amount depending only on T_1 and T_2;
(iii) The length of the final states of A_∞ equals 0.

From (6) we obtain a semialgorithm for the equivalence of T_1 and T_2. Since a semialgorithm for the nonequivalence is trivial our proof is complete. □

It follows immediately from the above proof that the theorem holds also in the case when the output structure is a finitely generated free group instead of such a monoid. Similar results, even in stronger forms, have been proved in [Li1] and [Li2]. If the determinism is defined like in deterministic pushdown automata, i.e., in a state it is allowed to read the empty word provided that in this state no symbol can be read, then we obtain a wider class of transducers. For this class the equivalence problem is shown to be decidable in [BH2].

Theorem 3 was generalized for single-valued transducers in [S] and independently in [BH1]:

<u>Theorem 4</u>. The equivalence problem for single-valued transducers is decidable.

Next step in generalizing Theorem 3 was made in [GI] where the following result was proved:

Theorem 5. The equivalence problem for finite-ambiguous transducers is decidable.

Still one step in generalizing the above decidability results for one-way transducers was achieved recently as a consequence of a more general result of [CK3]:

Theorem 6. $EP_{\forall}(FV1T, HDT0L)$ is decidable.

Outline of the proof. The proof is based on the following two important results: (i) The validity of the Ehrenfeucht Conjecture, which states that each system of equations over a finitely generated free monoid and with a finite number of unknowns is equivalent to its finite subsystem; cf. [K] and [AL1]. (ii) The decidability result of Makanin, which states that it is decidable whether a given equation over a finitely generated free semigroup has a solution, cf. [Mak].

In addition to these results we use techniques, cf. [CK2] or [CK3], which allow to state the fact that two considered transducers are equivalent on a given word in terms of solutions of certain systems of equations over a free monoid. In this way we associate languages with systems of equations. Further the languages we are considering, HDTOL languages, are in a certain sense morphically defined, and hence it turns out that the systems of equations associated with these languages are so simple that equivalent finite subsystems (guaranteed by the Ehrenfeucht Conjecture) can be effectively found.

The construction of the above systems of equations depends on the k-valuedness of the transducers. So we have to be able to find such a k. This can be done by a result in [GI] (assuming that, as is the case, the transducers are finite-valued).

□

Corollary 1. The equivalence problem for finite-valued transducers is decidable.

Now, it is interesting to compare Corollary 1 with Theorems 1 and 2. The characteristic feature of the transducers in Corollary 1 is that there exists an upper bound for the number of different outputs produced for single input words. Freely speaking this can be stated that the global degree of nondeterminism (with respect to outputs) is bounded. In this case the equivalence problem is decidable. On the other hand, if this degree of nondeterminism is unbounded, then the problem becomes undecidable even in quite restrictive cases as shown by Theorem 2.

On the previous lines we generalized Theorem 3 by allowing some nondeterminism. Another direction to generalize it is to consider more powerful deterministic transducers, for example two-way transducers. It was for a long time an open problem to decide whether two deterministic two-way transducers are equivalent, until it was solved by Gurari in [G1], cf. also [G2]:

Theorem 7. The equivalence problem for deterministic two-way transducers is decidable.

Recently this result was generalized in [CK2] as follows:

Theorem 8. The equivalence problem for single-valued two-way transducers is decidable.

The proof of Theorem 8 resembles that of Theorem 6, and in fact the same ideas can also be used to generalize it for k-valued or finite-valued two-way transducers, cf. [CK3].

4. Universal equivalence of mappings on languages

In this section we consider mappings which are compositions of morphisms and inverse morphisms and study the universal equivalence of such mappings on languages, mainly on regular languages. The problem of asking whether two morphisms are equivalent on a given language was first explicitly studied in [CS], although the same problem had occurred implicitly already earlier in connection with some other problems. Indeed, the well-known DOL sequence equivalence problem, cf. [CF] or [CK1], can be stated in this form as follows: given a word w in Σ^* and two morphisms h and g from Σ^* into itself decide whether h and g are equivalent on the language $\{h^n(w) \mid n \geq 0\}$.

Concerning morphisms the following result was proved in [CS], cf. also [ACK] and [I2] where the result has been generalized:

Theorem 9. $EP_{\forall}(H,CF)$ is decidable.

As an evidence of the nontriviality of our Theorem 6 we note that it contains as a special case the following result which, in turn, is a proper generalization of the above mentioned DOL sequence equivalence problem.

Theorem 10. $EP_{\forall}(H,HDT0L)$ is decidable.

Next we turn to consider more general mappings. Based on the fact that finite one-way transducers can be simulated by morphisms and inverse morphisms, cf. e.g. [KL], the following result was deduced from Theorem 1 in [KK]:

Theorem 11. $EP_{\forall}(HoH^{-1},Reg)$ is undecidable.

Actually, in Theorem 11 the family Reg can be replaced by the family $\mathcal{F} = \{F^* \mid F \text{ is finite}\}$. Consequently, we also have:

<u>Theorem 12</u>. $EP_\forall(\mathcal{H} \circ \mathcal{H}^{-1} \circ \mathcal{H}, \Sigma^*)$ is undecidable.

On the other hand, it was also shown in [KK] that if we reverse the order of morphisms and inverse morphisms, then the problem becomes decidable (ever for the family $\mathcal{CF}$ as shown in [Mao3]).

<u>Theorem 13</u>. $EP_\forall(\mathcal{H}^{-1} \circ \mathcal{H}, \text{Reg})$ is decidable.

Theorems 11 and 13 are interesting in the sense that they reveal the borderline between the decidability and the undecidability in a certain setting. More precisely, let us call a partial mapping <u>morphic</u> if it is a composition of morphisms and inverse morphisms. Now, Theorems 11 and 13 determine sharply for which types of compositions their equivalence on regular languages can be decided.

A natural way to generalize the notion of a morphism is to consider substitutions. In this case the most important decidability question is however unanswered:

<u>Open problem 1</u>. Is the $EP_\forall(\mathcal{S}, \text{Reg})$ decidable or not?

We feel that this problem is interesting, but also difficult. There exists some support for this evaluation. First of all it can be shown, cf. [AL2], that, not only for regular languages, but for all languages the following result holds: Given a natural number $k \geq 0$ and a language $L \subseteq \Sigma^*$, then there exists a finite subset F of L such that, for any two finite substitutions σ and τ satisfying $\max\{\text{card}(\sigma(a)), \text{card}(\tau(a)) \mid a \in \Sigma\} \leq k$, σ and τ are equivalent on L if and only if they are equivalent on F. So the question is whether such an F can be found effectively for each regular language. It would be surprising if this is not the case. On the other hand, the above result does not hold even noneffectively for the regular language ab^*a with respect to <u>all</u> finite substitutions as shown in [La].

Our conjecture is that $EP_\forall(\mathcal{S}, \text{Reg})$ is decidable. However, as the second evidence of its nontriviality we mention the following related result of [Mao2]:

<u>Theorem 14</u>. Given a regular language $L \subseteq \Sigma^*$ and two finite substitutions σ and τ on Σ^* it is undecidable whether the relation $\sigma(x) \subseteq \tau(x)$ holds for all x in L.

We conclude this section by stating a generalization of Theorem 11 due to [Mao1]:

Theorem 15. $EP_{\forall}(S^{-1},Reg)$ is undecidable.

5. Other types of equivalences and open problems

First we consider the existential equivalence. Intuitively it is clear that it is more difficult to decide the existential rather than the universal equivalence of two mappings. That this is really the case is seen from the following result proved in [KM], cf. Theorem 13:

Theorem 16. $EP_{\exists}(H^{-1},Reg)$ is undecidable.

Actually, Theorem 16 remains valid if, like in Theorem 11, Reg is replaced by F. Since the problem $EP_{\exists}(H,Reg)$ is trivially decidable, as a special case of that of Theorem 13, we have found also in the case of the existential equivalence of morphic mappings on regular languages a sharp borderline between the decidability and the undecidability.

Concerning the equivalence with multiplicities we have only the following simple observation (due to T. Harju): For any finite transducer T if we add to it, for each state q, the loops (q,λ,λ,q) we obtain a transducer which produces every output with the multiplicity ∞. Hence, the problem $EP_M(1T,\Sigma^*)$ is undecidable by Theorem 1. However, this undecidability is based on the identity $a+\infty=\infty$ and is thus in a sense artificial. So let us consider only such transducers which do not have any transitions in $Q\times\{\lambda\}\times\{\lambda\}\times Q$. Let us denote the family of such one-way transducers by $1T_e$. Obviously each transducer T in this class satisfies: the multiplicity of $y \in |T|(x)$, for any $x \in \Sigma^*$ and $y \in \Delta^*$, is bounded. On the other hand, it is also obvious that, for any one-way transducer T' satisfying this condition, there exists a transducer T" in $1T_e$ such that T' and T" are equivalent with multiplicities.

Now, we state

Open problem 2. Is the problem $EP_M(1T_e,\Sigma^*)$ decidable?

We again conjecture that this is the case, and further that the problem is difficult. Indeed, a solution to this problem would immediately give a solution to the equivalence problem for deterministic two-tape acceptors, which is known to be decidable, but not easy, cf. [Bi].

We conclude this paper by discussing more our first open problem $EP_{\forall}(S,Reg)$ introduced in Section 4. We give an equivalent formulation of this problem in terms of equivalence problems for transducers. In order to be able to do this we call a one-way transducer T input deterministic if the underlying automaton of T is deterministic. (So each input deterministic transducer is a gsm.) Let us denote this family of transducers by $\mathcal{D}_i 1T$. We have

Open problem 1'. Is the problem $EP_\forall(\mathcal{D}_i 1T, \Sigma^*)$ decidable?

Based on the well-known fact that the set of accepting computations of a finite automaton forms a regular set it is not difficult to prove, cf. [CK3]:

Theorem 17. The problem $EP_\forall(S, Reg)$ is decidable if and only if $EP_\forall(\mathcal{D}_i 1T, \Sigma^*)$ is decidable.

We feel that Theorem 17 makes our problem 1 even more interesting.

Acknowledgement. The author is grateful to T. Harju and E. Kinber for useful discussions.

References

[ACK] Albert, J., Culik II, K. and Karhumäki, J., Test sets for context-free languages and algebraic systems of equations, Inform. Control 52 (1982) 172-186.

[AL1] Albert, M. and Lawrence, J., A proof of Ehrenfeucht's conjecture, Theoret. Comput. Sci. 41 (1985) 121-123.

[AL2] Albert, M. and Lawrence, J., Test sets for finite substitutions, Theoret. Comput. Sci. 43 (1986) 117-122.

[Be] Berstel, J., Transductions and Context-Free Languages (Teubner Stuttgard, 1979).

[Bi] Bird, M., The equivalence problem for deterministic two-tape automata, J. Comput. System Sci. 7 (1973) 218-236.

[BH1] Blattner, M. and Head, T., Single-valued a-transducers, J. Comput. System Sci. 15 (1977) 310-327.

[BH2] Blattner, M. and Head, T., The decidability of equivalence for deterministic finite transducers, J. Comput. System Sci. 19 (1979) 45-49.

[CF] Culik II, K. and Fris, I., The decidability of the equivalence problem for DOL-systems, Inform. Control 35 (1977) 20-39.

[CK1] Culik II, K. and Karhumäki, J., A new proof for the DOL sequence equivalence problem and its implications, in A. Salomaa and G. Rozenberg (eds): The Book of L (Springer, Berlin, 1986).

[CK2] Culik II, K. and Karhumäki, J., The equivalence problem for single-valued two-way transducers (on NPDTOL languages) is decidable, SIAM J. of Comput. (to appear).

[CK3] Culik II, K. and Karhumäki, J., The equivalence of finite valued transducers (on HDTOL languages) is decidable, Proceedings of MFCS 86, Theoret. Comput. Sci. 47 (1986) 71-84.

[CS] Culik II, K. and Salomaa, A., On the decidability of morphic equivalence for languages, J. Comput. System Sci. 17 (1978) 163-175.

[E] Eilenberg, S., Automata, Languages and Machines, vol. A (Academic Press, New York, 1974).

[EY] Ehrich, R. and Yau, S., Two-way sequential transductions and stack automata, Inform. Control 18 (1971) 404-446.

[FR] Fischer, P. and Rosenberg, A., Multitape one-way nonwriting automata, J. Comput. System Sci. 2 (1968) 88-101.

[Gr] Griffiths, T., The unsolvability of the equivalence problem for ε-free nondeterministic generalized machines, J. Assoc. Comput. Mach. 15 (1968) 409-413.

[Gu1] Gurari, E., The equivalence problem for deterministic two-way transducers is decidable, SIAM J. Comput. 11 (1982) 448-452.

[Gu2] Gurari, E., Two-way counter machines and finite-state transducers, J. Comput. Math. 17 (1985) 229-236.

[GI] Gurari, E. and Ibarra, O., A note on finite-valued and finitely ambiguous transducers, Math. Systems Theory 16 (1983) 61-66.

[H] Harrison, M., Introduction to Formal Languages (Addison-Wesley, Reading, MA, 1978).

[I1] Ibarra, O., The unsolvability of the equivalence problem for ε-free NGSM's with unary input (output) alphabet and applications, SIAM J. Comput. 4 (1978) 524-532.

[I2] Ibarra, O., 2DST mappings on languages and related problems, Theoret. Comput. Sci. 19 (1982) 219-227.

[JL] Jones, N. and Laaser, W., Complete problems for deterministic polynomial time, Theoret. Comput. Sci. 3 (1977) 105-117.

[K] Karhumäki, J., The Ehrenfeucht Conjecture: A compactness claim for finitely generated free monoids, Theoret. Comput. Sci. 29 (1984) 285-308.

[KK] Karhumäki, J. and Kleijn, H.C.M., On the equivalence problem of compositions of morphisms and inverse morphisms, RAIRO Inform. Théor. 19 (1985) 203-211.

[KL] Karhumäki, J. and Linna, M., A note on morphic characterization of languages, Discrete Appl. Math. 5 (1983) 243-246.

[KM] Karhumäki, J. and Maon, Y., A simple undecidable problem: Existential egreement of inverses of two morphisms on a regular language, J. Comput. System Sci. 32 (1986) 315-322.

[La] Lawrence, J., The non-existence of finite test sets for set-equivalence of finite substitutions, EATCS Bull. 28 (1986) 34-37.

[Li1] Lisovik, L.P., Finite coverings of regular events by strong sets, Doklady of Ukrainian Academy of Sciences (1979) N 5.

[Li2] Lisovik, L.P., On solvable problems for Converters with Finite Rotary Counters, Kibernetika (1985) N 3 1-8.

[Mak] Makanin, G.S., The problem of solvability of equations in a free semigroup, Mat. Sb. 103 (1977) 147-236.

[Mao1] Maon, Y., On the equivalence of some transductions involving letter to letter morphisms on regular languages, manuscript (1985).

[Mao2] Maon, Y., Decision problems concerning equivalence of transductions on languages, Ph.D. Thesis, Tel Aviv University (1985).

[Mao3] Maon, Y., On the equivalence problem of composition of morphisms and inverse morphisms on context-free languages, manuscript (1984).

[Mo] Moore, E.F., Gedanken-experiments on sequential machines, in: Automata Studies (Princeton University Press, 1956).

[NRSS] Nielsen, M., Rozenberg, G., Salomaa, A. and Skyum, S., Nonterminals, homomorphisms and codings in different variations of OL systems. I and II, Acta Inform. 3 (1974) 357-364 and 4 (1974) 87-106.

[RS] Rozenberg, G. and Salomaa, A., The Mathematical Theory of L Systems (Academic Press, New York 1980).

[S] Schützenberger, M.P., Sur les relations rationelles in: Lecture Notes in Computer Science 33 (Springer, Berlin 1975) 209-213.

[SS] Salomaa, A. and Soittola, M., Automata-Theoretic Aspects of Formal Power Series (Springer, Berlin 1978).

KLEENE'S THEOREM REVISITED

Jacques Sakarovitch
Laboratoire d'Informatique Théorique et Programmation
C.N.R.S. et Université Paris VI
4, place Jussieu 75251 Paris Cedex 05, France

Abstract:The analysis of the famous Kleene's theorem shows that it consists indeed in two different propositions that are better distinguished when one tries to generatize the result. The first one relates rational expressions and a suitable generalization of finite automata. It holds in any monoid or, even better, in the semiring of formal power series on any monoid. It is shown that several classical results in formal language theory, for instance Elgot and Mezei characterization of rational relations by transducers and Chomsky normal form for context-free grammars, can thus be seen as particular cases of this first half of Kleene's theorem.

One of the basic results in automata theory is certainly the theorem of Kleene. It is presented in almost every textbook on the subject, it is taught in almost every academic cursus in computer science. In this conference I propose to study once again this fundamental result.

It is not surprising, but still noteworthy, that Kleene's Theorem has been given several equivalent statements and proved in several (slightly) different ways. Let us begin our investigations with a closer look at the two main versions of the theorem.

Most textbooks first define finite automata (either deterministic or non deterministic ones) on a finite input alphabet *A*. Any set of strings of elements of *A* — a *language* on *A* — accepted by a finite automaton is called *regular*. On the other hand three *regular operations* on languages are defined : the union and the product of two languages, and the Kleene's closure, or the star, of a language. And Kleene's Theorem is then stated the following way. *The class of regular languages* (i.e. the class of languages accepted by finite automata) *is the smallest class containing all finite sets and closed under regular*

operations (i.e. union, product, and star). The 1969 and 1979 editions of Hopcroft and Ullman's book [6,7] are good representatives of this version. In this presentation I could not help to point on what seems to me an awkwardness of the terminology : regular languages and regular operations are not related by a definition but by a result (Kleene's theorem indeed). It may also be noted that the original version of the result ([8], Theorems 3 and 4) uses the terminology that prevailed then : events instead of languages, nerve nets instead of finite automata, and the regular events were defined as those described by regular expressions.

Another version of Kleene's Theorem originated in the work of M. P. Schützenberger and of S. Eilenberg (we follow here the presentation given by J. Berstel in [1]). The idea is first to consider arbitrary monoids, instead of restricting oneself to free monoids (that are the set of strings over an alphabet), and then, given an arbitrary monoid M, to define two classes of subsets of M : the class of *recognizable* subsets of M, denoted by $\mathrm{Rec}\, M$ and the class of *rational* subsets of M, denoted by $\mathrm{Rat}\, M$. A subset of M is recognizable if it is an union of classes for a congruence of M of finite index. The class $\mathrm{Rat}\, M$ of rational sets of M is the smallest class containing the finite subsets and closed, as above, by these operations union, product, and star. Eilenberg has called these operations *rational*, rather than regular, to stress on the fact that the star operation is a kind of a formal inverse and that the generalization of rational sets to formal power series gives back the classical rational power series which are no new objects (and thus do not deserve a new name). I follow here this terminology. Kleene's Theorem is then stated as follows : if M is a finitely generated free monoid then both classes coincide, that is, if A is finite then $\mathrm{Rec}\, A^* = \mathrm{Rat}\, A^*$. The connection with the first version is easily made by the proof (often known as Nerode's Theorem) that a language of A^* is accepted by a finite automaton if, and only if, it is recognizable.

The framework that is set up to state this second version of Kleene's Theorem brings in several advantages. First, it is well suited — it was indeed devised for that purpose — to the generalization of the result from subsets of the free monoid to formal power series on the same free monoid and over any semiring of coefficients (in the beginning, only commutative semirings of coefficients were considered but this is an unnecessary restriction). Second, it helps to clarify the study of rational languages, allowing to distinguish between the properties that are due to recognizability and those that come with rationality. These properties extend respectively to recognizable and rational sets of non free monoids that are quite useful objects (e.g. rational relations, or semilinear sets). Let us also mention a third point which is of great value but somewhat outside the scope of this conference. Both rationality and recognizability are concepts that can be investigated in other structures than monoids or semirings of formal power series; they are concepts of universel algebra. In these general structures (think for instance of trees), both are ways to give finite descriptions of certain (simple) infinite sets of elements, which is the common task for mathematicians and for computer scientists, even if for the later "infinite" means only "very large".

In my opinion, the definition of the two classes Rat and Rec has had also a slight drawback. It has put some shadow on the fact that between Rat and Rec there is a natural bridge, or at least a bridge used by everyone, namely the finite automata, or a suitable generalization of those, which I call *mechanisms*, after J. H. Conway [3].

The aim of this conference is to make clear that Kleene's Theorem consists indeed in two distinct steps. The first one, called here the fundamental theorem on mechanisms, states that the class Rat is equal to the class of results of mechanisms (this will be more precisely defined later on). The important fact is that this results holds in *any monoid* or in *any semiring of formal power series* (over a suitable semiring of coefficients). The second step is the equality of the class Rec with the results of mechanisms in the case of finitely generated free monoids or of formal power series on these free monoids. This presentation of Kleene's Theorem is given in the first part.

The significance, or the usefulness, of this analysis of Kleene's Theorem should appear in the second part where it is sketched, on two examples, how the fundamental theorem on mechanisms is indeed the essence of several other basic results in automata and formal language theory. The two examples are the transducers characterization of rational relations by Elgot and Mezei, and the Chomsky normal form of context free grammars.

1 A two-step generalized Kleene's theorem

The purpose of this first part is to indicate the definitions and propositions that blaze the trail to Kleene Theorem. The first task is to define a sufficiently general structure which we call Kleene's semiring where the Kleene's closure, the star, can be defined. The second one is the more classical definition of formal power series on a monoid. We then define the mechanisms, the generalization of finite automata, which will play the central rôle in the proof.

The interested reader will find more details and developments, as well as the missing definitions, in [1],[2],or [4], and, for the new aspects, in [10]. The reader disheartened by what he thinks nonsensible bourbakism should keep in mind that the various generalizations considered here are just the necessary ones to reach context free grammars at the end of the work.

1.1 Kleene semi-ring

A monoid M is a set equipped with an associative operation and an identity that is denoted by 1_M. A semiring $\mathbf{K}$ is a set equipped with two operations : addition and multiplication. The addition makes of $\mathbf{K}$ a commutative monoid and the multiplication makes of $\mathbf{K}$ a (non necessarily commutative) monoid and is distributive over the addition; the identity for the addition, denoted 0, is a zero for the multiplication.

If M is a monoid, the set of subset of M denoted by $\mathcal{P}(M)$ is canonically equipped with the multiplication :

$$\forall P, R \in M \qquad PR = \{pr \mid p \in P, r \in R\}$$

Together with the union of sets, which will thus be denoted by $+$ instead of $\cup$, this multiplication gives to $\mathcal{P}(M)$ a structure of semiring. The subset $\{o, \{1_M\}\}$ of $\mathcal{P}(M)$ is isomorphic to the Boolean semiring $\mathbf{B} = \{0, 1\}$.

A semiring $\mathbf{K}$ is *complete* if any sum, even infinite, is defined on $\mathbf{K}$; (and if these infinite sums satisfy the obvious associativity and distributivity identities). For any monoid M, $\mathcal{P}(M)$ is a complete semiring.

A unary operator, the *star*, is defined on a complete semiring $\mathbf{K}$ by

$$\forall k \in K \qquad k^* = \sum_{n \in N} k^n$$

(with the conventions $k^0 = 1$ and $k^{n+1} = k^n k$).

The problem we are faced with is the definition of the star on semirings that are not necessarily complete. The method used by Conway in [3] leads to the following definitions. A semiring $\mathbf{K}$ is *ordered* if the relation $\leq$ defined by

$$\forall k, l \in \mathbf{K} \qquad k \leq l \qquad \Leftrightarrow \qquad \exists h \in \mathbf{K} \qquad k + h = l$$

is an ordering relation. An ordered complete semiring is *continuous* if, for any set I of indices, $\sum_{i \in I} k_i$ is the least upper bound of all the $\sum_{i \in J} k_i$ for any finite subset J of I. For any monoid M, $\mathcal{P}(M)$ is a continuous ordered complete semiring.

In the sequel, continuous semiring means continuous ordered complete semiring. A semiring $\mathbf{K}$ is called a *Kleene semiring* if it is a subsemiring of a continuous semiring and closed under star. For any monoid M, $\operatorname{Rat} M$ is a Kleene semiring but not a complete semiring.

PROPOSITION 1 .— *Let $\mathbf{K}$ be a Kleene semiring. For any k and h in $\mathbf{K}$, k^*h is the smallest solution of the equation $X = h + kX$.*

From which one deduces

PROPOSITION 2 .— *Let X be a square matrix the entries of which belong to a Kleene semiring. Then the entries of X^* are rational expressions of the entries of X.*

The proof of these two propositions are identical to those of Theorems 3.3 and 3.5 of [3].

1.2 Rational power series

A *formal power series* on a monoid M with coefficients in a semiring $\mathbf{K}$ is any mapping of M into $\mathbf{K}$ and can be represented as a formal sum of elements of M with coefficients in $\mathbf{K}$. We write

$$\forall s \in \mathbf{K}\langle\langle M\rangle\rangle \qquad s = \sum_{m \in M} < s, m > m$$

where $< s, m >$ is the coefficient of s on m.

If $\mathbf{B}$ is the Boolean semiring, then $\mathbf{K}\langle\langle M\rangle\rangle$ is equal to $\mathcal{P}(M)$; we keep the later notation.

Elements of $\mathbf{K}\langle\langle A^*\rangle\rangle$ are thus generalization of languages — first considered by M. P. Schützenberger in [1]. S. Eilenberg calls the formal power series *sets with multiplicity* and presents all the theory of (rational) languages in this setting [4]. One motivation for that generalization is the study of ambiguity. One is interested not only to know whether a word is accepted or not by an automaton but also by the number of computations of the automaton that lead to the acceptance of the word. Another motivation is that it allows uniform, and mathematically smoother, treatment of different objects like languages and relations.

The set $\mathbf{K}\langle\langle M\rangle\rangle$, equipped with the Cauchy product, is a semiring; the Cauchy product is well-defined either when $\mathbf{K}$ is complete, or when M is *graded* (A monoid is said to be graded if every element has only a finite number of distinct factorizations — in [4] "graded" is called *locally finite*). A free monoid is graded.

The connection between the properties of $\mathbf{K}$ and $\mathbf{K}\langle\langle M\rangle\rangle$ with respect to the star operation is given by :

Lemma 3 . — *If* $\mathbf{K}$ *is a continuous semiring, then* $\mathbf{K}\langle\langle M\rangle\rangle$ *is a continuous semiring. If* M *is graded and* $\mathbf{K}$ *a Kleene semiring then* $\mathbf{K}\langle\langle M\rangle\rangle$ *is a Kleene semiring.*

Example : if M is any monoid, $(\mathrm{Rat}\, M)\langle\langle A^*\rangle\rangle$ is a Kleene semiring.

In the sequel, it will always be assumed either that $\mathbf{K}$ is continuous, or that M is graded and $\mathbf{K}$ a Kleene semiring.

A power series with a finite number of non zero coefficient is a *polynomial.* The set of polynomials of $\mathbf{K}\langle\langle M\rangle\rangle$ is denoted by $\mathbf{K}\langle M\rangle$. Finaly, a power series of $\mathbf{K}\langle\langle M\rangle\rangle$ is *proper* if its coefficient on 1_M is zero.

The least subsemi-algebra of $\mathbf{K}\langle\langle M\rangle\rangle$ containing $\mathbf{K}\langle M\rangle$ and closed under the star operation is denoted by $\mathbf{K}\mathrm{Rat}\, M$; its elements are the $\mathbf{K}$*-rational* series on M. We have already used the notation $\mathrm{Rat}\, M$ when $\mathbf{K}$ is the Boolean semiring.

It should be noted this is *not* the classical definition of $(\mathbf{K}-)$ rational series which supposes the closure under star only for proper series. We loose here in generality but we gain in simplicity. A little more care makes it possible to unify both definitions (cf. [4,10]).

1.3 Mechanisms

Let us start from the classical definition of finite automata. A non deterministic finite automaton is a 5-tuple $\mathcal{A} = < Q, A, \delta, q_0, F >$ where Q is the (finite) set of states, A the input alphabet, $\delta : A \times Q \to \mathcal{P}(Q)$ the transition function, q_0 the initial state, and F the set of final states. Mechanisms are a double generalization of finite automata. In the definition of $\delta : Q \times A \to \mathcal{P}(Q)$ let us interpret A as a set of elements of the free monoid A^*. Roughly speaking we have a mechanism in full generality if we replace in the definition above A^* by any monoid M and the set A by any set of subsets of M. We find it convenient to use mechanisms by means of their *matrix representation* for it allows shorter and easier proofs (eventhough they may then appear as less intuitive proofs); we shall thus give the formal definition of mechanisms under this representation.

Before this, let us recall that finite automata also may be given a matrix representation. Let $\mathcal{A} = < Q, A, \delta, q_0, F >$ be a finite automaton. Let X be the $Q \times Q$-matrix with entries in $\mathcal{P}(A)$ defined by

$$X_{p,q} = \{a \in A \mid q \in \delta(p,a)\}$$

Let I be the Boolean row-vector and T the Boolean colum-vector, both of dimension Q, defined by

$$\begin{cases} I_q = 1 & \text{if } q = q_0 \\ \quad\; = 0 & \text{otherwise} \end{cases} \qquad \begin{cases} T_p = 1 & \text{if } p \in F \\ \quad\; = 0 & \text{otherwise} \end{cases}$$

The triple (I, X, T) is another description of the automaton $\mathcal{A}$ and it is known that $L(\mathcal{A})$, the language recognized by $\mathcal{A}$, is equal to the set IX^*T (cf. [4] for instance).

DEFINITION 1 .— *Let* $\mathbf{K}$ *be a semiring and* M *a monoid. Let* Q *be a finite set. A* mechanism over $\mathbf{K}\langle\langle M\rangle\rangle$ of dimension Q *is a triple* (I, X, T) *where* X *is a* $Q \times Q$*-matrix with entries in* $\mathbf{K}\langle\langle M\rangle\rangle$*, and where* I *and* T *are respectively a row-vector and a column-vector, both of dimension* Q*, with entries in* $\mathbf{K}$.

The *result* of a mechanism (I, X, T) is the series IX^*T. Two mechanisms are *equivalent* if they have the same result.

The matrix representation of finite automata goes back to the beginning of the theory of automata and may be considered as folklore. The name of mechanism was introduced by J. H. Conway who considered in [3] only mechanisms on free monoids and made a systematic use of the matrix representation. The generalized M-automata of [4] are mechanisms the entries of which are elements of M; the result of such a generalized M-automaton is either a subset of M, or a series in $\mathcal{N} \langle\langle M \rangle\rangle$, where $\mathcal{N}$ is the completion of $\mathbf{N}$, the set of integers, by an element infinity.

We can now state the fundamental theorem of mechanisms.

THEOREM 1 .— *Let* $\mathbf{K}$ *be a semiring,* M *a monoid, and* $\mathcal{C}$ *a generating set of* M*. Then* $\mathbf{K}\mathrm{Rat}\, M$ *is equal to the set of results of mechanisms the entries of which are in* $\mathcal{C}$.

The fact that the result of a mechanism is a rational expression of its entries is given by Proposition 2. The proof of the converse implication is identical to the classical proofs of Kleene's Theorem, basically by induction on the length of rational expressions. In [3] p.31, one finds such a proof that is written in the framework of matrix representations and that can be used verbatim.

Theorem 1 should not be thought as a generalized version of Kleene's Theorem. As was said in the introduction, it is rather the first half, the first step of Kleene's Theorem, which holds *in any monoid*. If Kleene's Theorem is said to be generalized here it is because it applies to formal power series instead of subsets of a free monoid. A generalization due to M. P. Schützenberger ([11]).

A last definition will be useful for the completion of Kleene's Theorem. A mechanism is said to be *proper* if its entries are proper. The fact that finite automata with "ε-moves" are equivalent to finite automata without ε-moves may be rephrased by te following :

LEMMA 4 . — *Any mechanism on M is equivalent to a proper mechanism on M.*

The proof of this lemma will demonstrate the power of the matrix representation. Let (I, X, T) be a mechanism over $\mathbf{K}\langle\langle M\rangle\rangle$. The matrix X may be uniquely written as $X = E + Y$ where E is a matrix over $\mathbf{K}$ and Y a proper matrix. We have

$$X^* = (E+Y)^* = (E^*Y)^*E^*$$

The entries of E^*Y are (finite) sums of the entries of Y; the mechanism (I, E^*Y, E^*T) it thus proper and equivalent to (I, X, T). ■

1.4 Kleene - Schützenberger Theorem

Since we already reached the fundamental theorem on mechanism which was our main goal we could stop here the first part. For sake of completeness, we sketch how one goes from mechanisms to recognizable power series, the second step of Kleene's Theorem. For that purpose we first define the recognizable power series.

Let $\mathbf{K}$ be a semiring and M a monoid. Let Q be a finite set. A $\mathbf{K}$-*automaton* on M of dimension Q is a triple (λ, μ, ν) where μ is a morphism from M into the square matrices of dimension Q over $\mathbf{K}$, and where λ and ν are respectively a row-vector and a column-vector both of dimension Q with entries in K.

$$\lambda \in \mathbf{K}^{1\times Q} \qquad \mu : M \to \mathbf{K}^{Q\times Q} \qquad \nu \in \mathbf{K}^{Q\times 1}$$

A series s of $\mathbf{K}\langle\langle M\rangle\rangle$ is *recognized*, or realized, or represented, by a $\mathbf{K}$-automaton (λ, μ, ν) if

$$s = \sum_{m\in M} (\lambda \cdot m\mu \cdot \nu) m$$

A series is *recognizable* if it is recognized by a K-automaton; the set of recognizable series of $\mathbf{K}\ll M\gg$ is denoted by $\mathbf{K}\mathrm{Rec}\,M$.

The connection with the classical (non deterministic) finite automata is straightforward. Let $\mathbf{K}$ be equal to $\mathbf{B}$, the Boolean semiring, and let M be equal to A^*. A morphism μ from A^* into $\mathbf{B}^{Q\times Q}$ is completely defined by the matrices $a\mu$ for a in A. Every matrix $a\mu$ defines a mapping from Q into $\mathcal{P}(Q)$ and conversely any mapping from Q into $\mathcal{P}(Q)$ defines a Boolean $Q\times Q$-matrix. Thus the set of matrices $a\mu$ defines a transition function for classical automaton with set of states Q and input alphabet A. The initial states are the elements q of Q such that $\lambda_q = 1$, the final states those for which $\nu_q = 1$. One then can state

Kleene-Schützenberger Theorem : *Let* $\mathbf{K}$ *be a semiring and* A *a finite alphabet. Then* $\mathbf{K}\mathrm{Rat}\,A^* = \mathbf{K}\mathrm{Rat}\,A^*$.

The proof goes as follow :

If s is in $\mathbf{K}\mathrm{Rec}\,A^*$,

then s is recognized by a K-automaton, by definition;

then s is the result of a mechanism over $\mathbf{K}\ll M\gg$, *because* A^* *is a free monoid*;

and the entries of this mechanism are in $\mathbf{K}<A^*>$, *because* A *is finite* ;

then s is in $\mathbf{K}\mathrm{Rat}\,M$, by Theorem 1 (or Proposition 2).

Conversely, if s is in $\mathbf{K}\mathrm{Rat}\,A^*$,

then s is the result of a mechanism on A^*, by Theorem 1 ;

and this mechanism may be chosen *proper*, by Lemma 4 ;

then this mechanism can be transformed into a K-automaton that recognizes s, *because* A^* *is a free monoid.* ■

In both parts of the proof the transition between proper mechanism and K-automaton is the consequence of the following (easy) lemma :

Lemma 5 . — *Let* $\mathbf{K}$ *be a semiring and* A *an alphabet. Let* Q *a finite set and* $\mu : A^* \to \mathbf{K}^{Q\times Q}$ *a morphism. Put* $X = \sum_{a\in A}(a\mu)a$. *Then, for every* f *in* A^*, $< X^*, f > = f\mu$.

It should be clear now that the version of Kleene's Theorem presented here uses exactly the same proofs than the others. These proofs may be seen as the fixed skeleton of Kleene's Theorem. The attention is drawn here on the body that can be build on the skeleton. A larger body is a hint for a stronger skeleton, and a deeper result.

2 Two applications of the fundamental theorem on mechanisms

As announced in the introduction, we present now two examples of classical results in automaton theory that are particular cases of Theorem 1 once the suitable framework has been set up. The first example deals with rational relations. It is quite straightforward. The second one is more involved. The prerequisite is the representation of pushdown automata by means of rational relations from the free monoid into the polycyclic monoid, a theory of interest by its own and that we shall sketch briefly.

2.1 Rational relations and finite transducers

Let A^* and B^* be two free monoids. A relation τ from A^* into B^* is defined by its graph $\hat{\tau}$, a subset of $A^* \times B^*$. The relation τ is said to be *rational* if $\hat{\tau}$ is a rational subset of the (non free) monoid $A^* \times B^*$. Rational relations are a widely used class of fundamental transformations, both from the theoretical point of view (classification of formal languages, subfamilies of context free languages cf. [1]) and from the practical point of view (syntactic analysis, search procedures in dictionaries, decoding theory). Rational relations were first defined by Elgot and Mezei ([5]), and characterized then as the relations realized by (finite) transducers. This characterization is an instancy of Theorem 1.

A *transducer* $\mathcal{T}$ from A^* into B^*, $\mathcal{T} = (Q, E, Q_-, Q_+)$, consists in a labelled graph (Q, E) where Q is a finite set of vertices (called states to stick with the terminology of automata theory), and where $E = Q \times A^* \times B^* \times Q$ is a *finite* set of labelled edges — the label of an edge is an element (x, y) of $A^* \times B^*$ — together with two distinguished subsets Q_- and Q_+ of Q : the sets of initial and final states respectively. The graph of the relation τ from A^* into B^* realized by $\mathcal{T}$ is by definition the set of pairs (f, g) that are the label of a path in (Q, E) starting in Q_- and terminating in Q_+.

The connection between transducers from A^* into B^* and mechanisms over $\mathcal{P}(A^* \times B^*)$ is immediate. A transducer $\mathcal{T} = (Q, E, Q_-, Q_+)$ defines the mechanism (I, X, T) of dimension Q by

$$\begin{cases} I_q &= 1 \text{ if } q \in Q_- \\ &= 0 \text{ otherwise} \end{cases} \qquad \begin{cases} T_p &= 1 \text{ if } p \in Q_+ \\ &= 0 \text{ otherwise} \end{cases}$$

and $X_{p,q} = \{(x, y) \mid (p, x, y, q) \in E\}$. The result of (I, X, T) is exactly the graph the relation realized by $\mathcal{T}$. Conversely any mechanism (I, X, T) over $\mathcal{P}(A^* \times B^*)$ with finite entries defines a transducer from A^* into B^* by using the same equalities.

Now Theorem 1 states that a relation realized by a transducer is rational and that conversely any rational relation from A^* into B^* can be realized by a transducer the edges of which are labelled by elements of the generating set $\mathcal{C}$ of $A^* \times B^*$:

$$\mathcal{C} = \{(a, 1) \mid a \in A\} \cup \{(1, b) \mid b \in B\}$$

and this is exactly the result of Elgot and Mezei.

2.2 Context free languages and rationality

As rational relations from a free monoid into another one, context free languages are objects of fundamental interest from both theoretical and practical points of view in computer science. Since they form a strict superset of rational languages, the connection between context free languages and rational sets cannot be done inside the free monoids ; it necessarily takes place in a multiplicative structure that is, roughly said, powerful enough to express the computations involved for their recognition. This connection will be sketched now and we will see how a classical result like Chomsky normal form finds naturally its place in this framework. A complete theory of context free languages within this framework, that has its origins in the work of Nivat ([9]) and Shamir ([12]), will be presented in [10]. The reader is supposed to be familiar with the classical definitions, notations and results of context free languages theory.

Let first Y be a finite alphabet and $\tilde{Y} = Y \cup \overline{Y}$ the "symmetrized" of Y : $\overline{Y}$ is disjoint from, and in a one-to-one correspondence with Y. Let Σ be the set of relations on $\tilde{Y}^*$ defined by

$$\Sigma = \begin{cases} y\bar{y} = 1 & \forall y \in Y \\ y\bar{z} = 0 & \forall y, z \in Y \quad y \neq z \end{cases}$$

The quotient of $\tilde{Y}^*$ by the congruence generated by Σ is called the *polycyclic monoid* generated by Y and denoted by $P(Y)$; the canonical morphism from $\tilde{Y}^*$ onto $P(Y)$ is denoted by ρ. Let us remark first that the relations Σ, and thus the multiplication in $P(Y)$, are a model for the behaviour of a pushdown stack. The letter y is interpreted as : "push the letter y in the stack" and the letter $\bar{y}$ as : "pop the letter y from the stack". The two kinds of relations in Σ express first that "push and pop y" is equivalent to doing nothing and second that "push y and pop z" is impossible if y is different from z. Note also that $(1_{P(Y)})\rho^{-1}$, the set of words of $\tilde{Y}^*$ that are equivalent to $1_{P(Y)}$ modulo the congruence generated by Σ, is the celebrated (one-sided, or semi) Dyck set. I then propose the following definition :

A language L of A^* is context free if, and only if, there exists an alphabet Y and a rational relation θ from A^* into $P(Y)$ such that $L = (1_{P(Y)})\theta^{-1}$.

This definition is not as surprising as it may look. Up to tiny technical details, and modulo a characterization of rational relations by means of morphisms and intersection with rational languages (cf.[1,4,9]), this definition is equivalent to the theorem of Chomsky - Schützenberger, and thus consistent with the classical definition.

Direct computations show that both context free grammars and pushdown automata yield rational relations from a free monoid into a polycyclic monoid that give the corresponding generated or accepted languages. Conversely Theorem 1 states that any rational relation θ from a free monoid A^* into a polycyclic monoid $P(Y)$ is the result of a mechanism (I, X, T) of dimension Q the entries of which are finite unions of elements of one of the three sets :

$$C_1 = \{(a, 1) \mid a \in A\}$$

$$C_2 = \{(1, y) \mid y \in Y\}$$
$$C_3 = \{(1, \bar{y}) \mid y \in Y\}$$

since $C = C_1 \cup C_2 \cup C_3$ is a generating set of $A^* \times P(Y)$. To the mechanism (I, X, T) corresponds a pushdown automaton $\mathcal{A}$ with set of states Q, input alphabet A, pushdown alphabet Y, and the following transition function δ :

if $(a, 1) \in X_{p,q}$ then $(q, y) \in \delta(p, a, y)$ for any y in Y — that is if $\mathcal{A}$ is in the state p and reads the letter a it goes to the state q, independantly of the topmost symbol of the stack and without changing the stack ;

if $(1, y) \in X_{p,q}$ then $(q, zy) \in \delta(p, 1, z)$ for any z in Y — that is if $\mathcal{A}$ is in the state p, it goes by an ε-move in the state q and write y on the stack ;

and if $(1, \bar{y}) \in X_{p,q}$ then $(q, 1) \in \delta(p, 1, y)$ — that is if $\mathcal{A}$ is in the state p with y at the top of the stack, it goes to the state q and erases y on the stack by an ε-move.

Thus Theorem 1 states that any context free language is accepted by a pushdown automaton of this very peculiar form. If one applies to the automaton $\mathcal{A}$ we have just defined the classical construction of a context free grammar equivalent to a pushdown automaton one gets a grammar G with $N = Q \times Y \times Q$ as set of nonterminals and with the set of productions P defined as follows :

$$\begin{array}{lll} (a,1) \in X_{p,q} & \Rightarrow \quad (p,y,r) \to a(q,y,r) \in P & \forall y \in Y \ \ \forall q \in Q \\ (1,y) \in X_{p,q} & \Rightarrow \quad (p,z,s) \to (q,y,r)(r,z,s) \in P & \forall z \in Y \ \ \forall r,s \in Q \\ (1,\bar{y}) \in X_{p,q} & \Rightarrow \quad (p,y,q) \to 1 \in P & \end{array}$$

Thus G is in Chomsky normal form, as we wanted. ■

REFERENCES

1. J. Berstel, *Transductions and Context free Languages*, Teubner, 1979.

2. J. Berstel, Ch. Reutenauer, *Les séries rationnelles et leurs languages*, Masson, 1984.

3. J. H. Conway, *Regular Algebra and Finite Machines*, Chapman and Hall, 1971.

4. S. Eilenberg, *Automata, languages, and Machines*, Vol. A, Academic Press, 1974.

5. C. C. Elgot and G. Mezei, On relations defined by generalized finite automata, *I.B.M. J. of Res. and Dev.* 9, 1965, 47 - 65.

6. J. E. Hopcroft and J. D. Ullman, *Introduction to Automata Theory, Languages and Computation*, Addison Wesley, 1979.

7. J. E. Hopcroft and J. D. Ullman, *Formal Languages and their relation to Automata*, Addison Wesley, 1969.

8. S. C. Kleene, Representation of Events in Nerve Nets and Finite Automata, in *Automata Studies* (C. E. Shannon and J. Mc Carty, Eds), Princeton University Press , 1956, 3-41.

9. M. Nivat, Transductions des languages de Chomsky, *Ann. Inst. Fourier* 18, 1968, 336-456.

10. J. Sakarovitch, *Théorie des Automates*, en préparation.

11. M. P. Schützenberger, Certain elementary families of automata, in *Proceedings of Symposium on Mathematical Theory of Automata*, Polytechnic Institute of Brooklyn, 1962, 139-153.

12. E. Shamir, A representation theorem for algebraic and context free power series in non commuting variables, *Inform. and Control* 11, 1967, 234-254.

SOME COMBINATORIAL PROBLEMS CONCERNING FINITE LANGUAGES

Zsolt Tuza
Computer and Automation Institute
Hungarian Academy of Sciences
H-1111 Budapest, Kende u. 13-17, Hungary

Abstract Some combinatorial functions are introduced for finite languages. Various conjectures and problems are raised.

0. INTRODUCTION

Finite structures have several applications in the theory of computers. The study of finite languages, however, is a relatively new field in formal language theory. Though powerful methods have been developed for handling classical Chomsky-type languages, they are not always suitable for providing sufficient information about the finite case. So it seems quite natural for us to apply combinatorial ideas when finite languages are considered.

On one hand, finite languages can be viewed as hypergraphs. In this way, some results of hypergraph theory can be interpreted for finite languages, and some of them can be extended for the infinite case also. On the other hand, grammars have a rich structure even if they generate finite languages; for example, graphs (i.e., 2-uniform hypergraphs) have not proved to be powerful enough for handling languages of length 2 (see e.g. [12]). These facts indicate the importance of developing new methods that should be built on a base involving combinatorial and algebraic ideas simultaneously.

In this paper we raise some problems related to combinatorial properties of finite languages. In Section 1, some basic notions of hypergraph theory are extended for finite languages. In Section 2 we define saturated languages, and in Section 3 we raise some problems concerning complexity.

Undefined notions can be found in [10] and [1].

1. COVERING AND INDEPENDENCE

Let L be a collection of finite languages. For convenience, we assume L is closed under complementation in the following weak sense: If $L_1, L_2 \in L$ and $L_1 \subsetneq L_2$ then $L_2 \setminus L_1 \in L$. Let $L_o \subsetneq L$ be a given subcollection of languages. (An interesting particular case occurs when L_o consists of just one language L_o). For any $L \in L$ we introduce the following definitions that are natural extensions of standard hypergraph theoretic notions. Throughout, $L_1 \cong L_2$ means there is a one-to-one mapping φ from the alphabet of L_1 to the alphabet of L_2, such that $w \in L_1$ if and only if $\varphi(w) \in L_2$. The number of words in L is denoted by $|L|$.

Transversal. An $L' \subseteq L$, $L' \in L$ is an L_o-*transversal* of L if for every $L_o \in L_o$ and $L'_o \subseteq L$, $L_o \cong L'_o$, we have $L' \cap L'_o \neq \emptyset$. The L_o-*transversal number*, denoted by $\tau(L, L_o, L)$ (or $\tau(L)$ when L and L_o are understood), is the minimum number of words in an L_o-transversal L' of L.

Independence. An $L' \subsetneq L$, $L' \in L$ is L_o-*independent* if there are no $L_o \in L_o$ and $L'_o \subseteq L'$ with $L_o \cong L'_o$. The L_o-*independence number* $\alpha(L) = \alpha(L, L_o, L)$ is the maximum number of words in an L_o-independent $L' \subseteq L$.

Packing. A collection $\{L_1, \ldots, L_t\}$ of languages is an L_o-*packing* in L if for every i, $1 \leq i \leq t$, $L_i \subseteq L$ and there is an $L'_i \in L_o$ with $L_i \cong L'_i$; moreover, $L_i \cap L_j = \emptyset$ for all i and j, $1 \leq i < j \leq t$. The L_o-*packing number* $\nu(L) = \nu(L, L_o, L)$ is the maximum number of languages L_i in an L_o-packing.

Covering. A collection $\{L_1, \ldots, L_t\}$ of languages is an L_o-*covering* of L if $L_1 \cup \ldots \cup L_t = L$ and for every i, $1 \leq i \leq t$, either $|L_i| = 1$ or there is an $L'_i \in L_o$ with $L_i \cong L'_i$. The L_o-*covering number* $\rho(L) = \rho(L, L_o, L)$ is the minimum number of languages L_i in an L_o-covering of L.

Decomposition. A collection $\{L_1, \ldots, L_t\}$ of languages is an L_o-*decomposition* of L if it is an L_o-covering and $L_i \cap L_j = \emptyset$ for all i and j, $1 \leq i < j \leq t$. The L_o-*decomposition number* $\rho^*(L) = \rho^*(L, L_o, L)$ is the minimum number of languages L_i in an L_o-decomposition of L.

There are some obvious inequalities between the parameters introduced above. Clearly, $\rho(L) \le \rho^*(L)$ and $\nu(L) \le \tau(L)$ for all L, L and L_o; also if $L_o = \{L_o\}$ then $\tau(L) \le |L_o|\nu(L)$. Moreover, since every transversal $L' \subseteq L$ yields an independent $L'' = L \setminus L'$ and vice versa, a result of Gallai [4] can be formulated for finite languages also.

Proposition 1.1. For every L, L and L_o, $\alpha(L,L_o,L) + \tau(L,L_o,L) = |L|$.

It can be shown that the problem of determining $\alpha(L)$, $\tau(L)$,... is NP-complete. Hence, it is an interesting question how tight estimates can be given for them. In particular, find fairly good upper bounds on the transversal and covering number, provided that L or L_o satisfies some assumptions.

For simplicity, at the moment we assume $L_o = \{L_o\}$. In the same way as the main results of [7], the following statement can be proved.

Theorem 1.2. If L_o contains words of at least two distinct lengths then $\rho(L,L_o,L) \le \alpha(L,L_o,L)$ holds for all L and L.

Trivially, the inequality $\rho(L) \le \alpha(L)$ is sharp when $L_o' \not\subseteq L$ for all $L_o' \cong L_o$. There are several examples, however, of languages L_o (of fixed length) for which there is an infinite sequence $L_1, L_2, \ldots$ of languages satisfying $\lim_{n\to\infty} \rho(L_n) / \alpha(L_n) = \infty$.

Problem 1.3. Characterize those L_o and L for which
(a) $\rho(L) \le \alpha(L)$ for all $L \in L$,

(b) $\rho^*(L) \le \alpha(L)$ for all $L \in L$.

If L is the class of symmetric languages of length 2 then the results of [7] yield the following characterization in case (a): An $L_o \in L$ satisfies (a) if and only if its alphabet Σ cannot be partitioned into two parts Σ_1 and Σ_2 such that each word $w \in L_o$ contains one element of Σ_1 and one of Σ_2.

For some other L and L_o, sufficient conditions follow from results of Lehel [6]. There is very little known, however, about decompositions (part (b) of the problem). Another equality due to Gallai involves ρ^* and can be formulated as follows.

Proposition 1.4. For every $L, \mathcal{L}$ and $\mathcal{L}_o = \{L_o\}$,
$\rho^*(L,L_o,\mathcal{L}) + (|L_o|-1)\,\nu(L,L_o,\mathcal{L}) = |L|$.

As a consequence of Propositions 1.1 and 1.4, $\alpha + \tau = \rho^* + (|L_o|-1)\nu$. Hence, inequalities involving decomposition and independence numbers can be formulated for transversal and packing numbers.

Let us raise a problem which is an improvement of the trivial upper bound $\tau \leq |L_o|\nu$, in a rather simple particular case.

Conjecture 1.5. Let $\mathcal{L}$ be the class of languages of length 2, and let $L_o = \{ab,ac,bc\}$. Then, for every $L \in \mathcal{L}$, $\tau(L,L_o,\mathcal{L}) \leq 2\nu(L,L_o,\mathcal{L})$.

It would also be interesting to prove Conjecture 1.5 for anti-symmetric languages (i.e., when $ab \in L$ implies $ba \notin L$), as well as its symmetric version (when $ab \in L$ implies $ba \in L$, and the words ba, ca, cb are added to L_o). For the symmetric case, some results are given in [15].

Another interesting question occurs when $L_o = \{ab,bc,ca\}$. Then the situation $\tau(L) = \nu(L)$ can be characterized. (More precisely, those L can be described in which $\tau(L') = \nu(L')$ for all $L' \subseteq L$.) Call $L_1, L_2, \ldots, L_k, L_{k+1} = L_1$ an L_o-cycle of length k if $|L_i \cap L_{i+1}| = 1$ for $1 \leq i \leq k$ and $L_i \cap L_j = \emptyset$ for $|i-j| > 1$. Among others, the following result is proved in [16].

Theorem 1.6. Let $L_o = \{ab,bc,ca\}$ and $\mathcal{L}$ be the class of languages of length 2. Then $\tau(L,L_o,\mathcal{L}) = \nu(L,L_o,\mathcal{L})$ for every L not containing odd L_o-cycles of length greater than 3.

Note that if L is an odd L_o-cycle of length ≥ 3 then $\tau(L) > \nu(L)$.

2. SATURATED LANGUAGES

Denote by $\mathcal{L}(n,k)$ the collection of languages of length k over an n-element alphabet, and set $\mathcal{L}(k) = \bigcup_n \mathcal{L}(n,k)$. From now on we assume $\mathcal{L} \subseteq \mathcal{L}(k)$ for some fixed k. For simplicity, if there is an $L' \subseteq L$ with $L' \cong L_o$, we write $L_o \subset L$ (and here $L_o = L$ is allowed).

Let $L_o \in \mathcal{L}(k)$ be a fixed language. Call an $L \in \mathcal{L} \subseteq \mathcal{L}(k)$ L_o-*saturated* if $L_o \not\subset L$ and $L_o \subset L'$ for all $L' \in \mathcal{L}$, $L \subsetneq L'$, $L' \neq L$. Define

$$\mathrm{sat}(n,L_o) = \mathrm{sat}(n,L_o,\mathcal{L}) = \min\{|L| : L \in \mathcal{L} \cap \mathcal{L}(n,k),\ L \text{ is } L_o\text{-saturated}\}.$$

Now the problem is to find the value of $\mathrm{sat}(n,L_o)$ and to describe the structure of languages that are L_o-saturated for a given $L_o \in L(k)$.

Conjecture 2.1. For every $L_o \in L(k)$, $sat(n,L_o) \leq O(n^{k-1})$.

For $k = 2$, the conjecture can be proved.

Theorem 2.2. If $L_o \in L(2)$ then $sat(n,L_o) \leq cn$ for some constant $c = c(L_o)$.

Moreover, the validity of Conjecture 2.1 for the restricted class of symmetric languages of length 2 has been established by Kászonyi and the author [5].

In fact, we have a conjecture stronger than 2.1 which, for k = 2, can be formulated in the following way.

Conjecture 2.3. For every $L_o \in L(2)$ there is a constant $c = c(L_o)$ such that $sat(n,L_o) = cn + o(n)$.

Recently, the symmetric version of Conjecture 2.2 has been proved by Truszczyński and the author [11] for the case when $\liminf_{n\to\infty} sat(n,L_o)/n$ is small. Further results for symmetric particular cases have been achieved by Erdős, Hajnal and Moon [3], Mader [8] and Ollman [9]; see also [5].

We note that saturated languages (as well as the function $sat(n,L_o)$) can be defined in a more general way. Details and further related problems are discussed in [13].

3. COMPLEXITY

For a finite language L, let G_L be the collection of context-free grammars generating L. Let prod(G) denote the number of productions in the grammar G, and define the complexity of L as $c(L) = \min\{prod(G): G \in G_L\}$. The problem of determining c(L) was raised by Bucher et al. [2]. Note that the complexity of L can be defined similarly for any class of languages and for any complexity measure.

In [12] we have proved $c(L) \leq O(n^2/\log n)$ for all $L \in L(n,2)$. This result can be generalized for languages of length k as follows.

Theorem 3.1. For every $L \in L(n,k)$, $c(L) \leq O(n^k/\log n)$.

The proof of this upper bound is based on the existence of decompositions of L into some languages that can be generated easily.

Remark 3.2. If $\{L_1,\dots,L_t\}$ is a covering of L then

$$c(L) \le \sum_{i=1}^{t} c(L_i).$$

Certainly, some languages have a very simple structure and can be generated easily. For example, let A and B be two finite non-empty sets. Then the language $L(A,B) = \{ab: a\in A,\ b\in B\}$ can be generated by $|A|+|B|$ regular productions. Though the languages $L(A,B)$ are very simple, their family is rich enough for proving $c(L) \le O(n^2/\log n)$ for $L\in \mathcal{L}(n,2)$. (It can be shown by a probabilistic argument that this upper bound is sharp, see [12].) It is quite natural now to raise the folloiwng question.

Problem 3.3. Find a reasonably simple family $\mathcal{L}_o \subseteq \bigcup_n \mathcal{L}(n,k)$ with the property that for every $L\in\mathcal{L}(n,k)$ there is an $\mathcal{L}_o$-covering $\{L_1,\dots,L_t\}$ with $c(L) \le c_o \sum_{i=1}^{t} c(L_i)$, where c_o is a constant (possibly depending on k but independent on n).

Though the properties of a "reasonably simple family" have not been described explicitly, the languages L(A,B) may undoubtedly belong to such an $\mathcal{L}_o \subseteq \bigcup \mathcal{L}(n,2)$. As a more general example, one can take $m \ge 2$ non-empty sets $A_1,\dots,A_m$ and define $L(A_1,\dots,A_m) = \{a_ia_j : a_i\in A_i,\ a_j\in A_j,\ 1 \le i < j \le m\}$.

It is not obvious that the family of all languages $L(A_1,\dots,A_m)$ can provide better coverings (in the sense of Problem 3.3) than that of all L(A,B) or even the collection of all $L(A_1,\dots,A_m)$ with the restriction $m \le m_o$ (where m_o is fixed). To formulate this property more precisely, set $\mathcal{L}_s = \{L\in \bigcup \mathcal{L}(n,2) : L = L(A_1,\dots,A_m)$ for some $m \le s\}$ and denote $L(m) = \{a_ia_j : 1 \le i < j \le m\}$ where $a_1,\dots,a_m$ are distinct elements of an alphabet. It is easily seen that $c(L(m)) = O(m)$ as $m \to \infty$. On the other hand, a theorem proved in [14] implies the following result.

Theorem 3.4. If $\{L_1,\dots,L_t\}$ is an $\mathcal{L}_s$-covering of L(m) then

$$\sum_{i=1}^{t} c(L_i) \ge m \log m/\log s.$$

Hence, the complexity of L(m) has a smaller order than that of any $\mathcal{L}_s$-decomposition of L(m) (if s is fixed).

At the end, let us raise one more problem related to complexity.

Problem 3.5. Let $L_o \in \mathcal{L}(n,k)$ be fixed. Determine

(a) $\max\{c(L) : L \in \mathcal{L}(n,k),\ L_o \not\subset L\}$, and

(b) $\max\{c(L) : L \in \mathcal{L}(n,k),\ L$ is L_o-saturated$\}$.

Since $c(L) \leq |L|$, the assumption $L_o \not\subset L$ sometimes implies that $c(L)$ is much smaller than $O(n^k/\log n)$, because $|L|$ is small. It would be interesting to see some examples of L_o for which the answer to (b) is considerably smaller than to (a). (An L_o-saturated language L is "sparse" as $L_o \not\subset L$, but it is filled with sublanguages that are almost isomorphic to L_o; hence, it would not be very surprising if a covering of L existed for which Remark 3.2 could be applied.)

Acknowledgement. I am grateful to *E. Csuhaj-Varju* for her helpful remarks and suggestions concerning an early version of this paper.

REFERENCES

1. C. Berge, Graphs and Hypergraphs, North-Holland, 1973.

2. W. Bucher, K. Culik II, H. Maurer and D. Wotschke, Concise description of finite languages, Theoretical Computer Sci. 14 (1981) 227-246.

3. P. Erdős, A. Hajnal and J.W. Moon, A problem in graph theory, Amer. Math. Monthly 71 (1964) 1107-1110.

4. T. Gallai, Über extreme Punkt- und Kantenmengen, Ann. Univ. Sci. Budapest Eötvös Sect. Math. 2 (1959) 133-138.

5. L. Kászonyi and Zs. Tuza, Saturated graphs with minimal number of edges, J. Graph Theory 10 (1986) 203-210.

6. J. Lehel, Covers in hypergraphs, Combinatorica 2 (1982) 305-309.

7. J. Lehel and Zs. Tuza, Triangle-free partial graphs and edge covering theorems, Discrete Math. 39 (1982) 59-65.

8. W. Mader, 1-Faktoren in Graphen, Math. Ann. 201 (1973) 269-282.

9. L.T. Ollman, $K_{2,2}$-saturated graphs with a minimal number of edges, in: Proc. 3rd South-East Conference on Combinatorics, Graph Theory and Computing, pp. 367-392.

10. A. Salomaa, Formal Languages, Academic Press, 1973.

11. M. Truszczyński and Zs. Tuza; Asymptotic results on saturated graphs, submitted.

12. Zs. Tuza, On the context-free production complexity of finite languages, Discrete Applied Math., to appear.

13. Zs. Tuza, A generalization of saturated graphs for finite languages, MTA SZTAKI Studies 185/1986, pp. 287-293.

14. Zs. Tuza, Intersection properties and extremal problems for set systems, in: Irregularities of Partitions, Proc. Colloq. Math. Soc. János Bolyai, Fertőd (Hungary) 1986, to appear.

15. Zs. Tuza, A conjecture on triangles of graphs, in preparation.

16. Zs. Tuza, Perfect triangle families, in preparation.

Chapter 2

THEORY OF FORMAL GRAMMARS

A CONNECTION BETWEEN DESCRIPTIONAL COMPLEXITY OF CONTEXT-FREE GRAMMARS AND GRAMMAR FORM THEORY

Erzsébet Csuhaj-Varjú
Computer and Automation Institute, Hungarian Academy of Sciences
H-1132 Budapest,Victor Hugo u. 18-22.
Hungary

1. INTRODUCTION

Descriptional complexity of languages is an important part of formal language theory. Results concerning the size of grammars and languages have not only theoretical importance but give useful techniques in proving other types of properties. Especially, results concerning normal forms - grammars being in simple forms and generating a whole class of languages- are of interest.The most well-known descriptional complexity measures of context-free grammars are **Var**,**Prod**,**Lev**, and **Hei**, that is the number of nonterminals,the number of productions,the number of grammatical levels and the length of the longest way in the digraph of grammatical levels,respectively.A descriptional complexity measure of a language, generated by grammars from a class of grammars, is defined as the minimum of the complexities of those grammars, from the grammar class, which generate the language. These notions were introduced by Gruska in 1967 ([G1]) and in 1969 ([G2]). He stated the basic results concerning the behaviour of these measures on the class of context-free languages in [G2] and [G3].Descriptional complexities of normal form grammar classes were studied by Kelemenová (see [K1],[K2],[K3]).

Another important area of formal language theory is the theory of structurally similar grammars,that is grammar form theory.Here similarity is defined via a special finite substitution of nonterminals and terminals in the form grammar. Nonterminals are substituted by pairwise disjoint finite sets of nonterminals and terminals by finite sets of terminal words (general interpretation) or by pairwise disjoint finite sets of terminals (strict interpretation). Properties of these similarity classes have been an exhaustively investigated area of language theory (see [W]).The degree of similarity of a grammar in the grammar family can be characterized by the notion of a bounded interpretation (see [C],[D],[CD]). Here the cardinality of the image of every nonterminal (terminal) is bounded by the same natural number.

The aim of this paper is twofold: first, we generalize some well-known results, as we show that complexity measures **Var**,**Lev**,**Hei**, and **Prod** are **unbounded** not only on the whole class of ε-free context-free languages but on all ε-free **subclasses** of ε-free context-free languages which are **similarity classes** (general or strict grammatical families) with respect to any corresponding similarity grammar class, that is general or strict grammar family, producing them.Second, we show that the **three area of language theory, that is, decriptional complexity, grammar form theory and normal form theory** are in close **connection**, as the **Var-complexity** of a context-free language with respect to a normal form grammar class (in the sense of [W]), that is to a strict grammar family of a special two-symbol grammar form, is **equal** to the **measure of boundness** of the interpretation which defines the **Var**-minimal grammar for the language from the grammar form. Moreover,we show that for every natural number n, for every normal form grammar class **F**, for every descriptional complexity measure **K**, where **K**$\in$\{**Lev**,**Hei**,**Var**,**Prod**\}, there is an ε-free context-free language L_K such that its K-complexity , with respect to **F**, is equal to n.

2. PRELIMINARIES

We first recall some basic notions. For further details the reader is referred to [C],[CD],[G2], [G3], [K1], [K2],[K3], [S],[W].

We use G=(N,T,P,S) for **context-free grammars** (shortly CF-grammars),where N is the set of nonterminals, T is the set of terminals, P is the set of productions and S is the startsymbol. L(G) denotes the **language** generated by G.

For a language L, alph(L) denotes the smallest alphabet Σ such that $L \subseteq \Sigma^*$ holds. For a word $w \in L$ lg(w) denotes the length of w.

We denote the class of context-free grammars, context-free languages, ε-free context-free grammars and ε-free languages by CF, CF^{ε}, L(CF), $L^{\varepsilon}(CF)$, respectively.

Here we consider **completely reduced** grammars. A context-free grammar G=(N,T,P,S) is said to be completely reduced iff for every $X \in N$ there is a $w \in T^*$ such that $X \overset{*}{\Rightarrow} w$ and there are $u,v \in (N \cup T)^*$ such that $S \overset{*}{\Rightarrow} uXv$ and G does not contain ε-rules and chain rules.
The class of completely reduced grammars is denoted by R.

A nonterminal X of G is said to be **recursive** iff there is a derivation $S \overset{*}{\Rightarrow} uXv \overset{*}{\Rightarrow} upXsv \overset{*}{\Rightarrow} w$ in G such that $u,v,p,s \in (N \cup T)^*$ and $ps \neq \varepsilon$. The set of recursive nonterminals of G is denoted by r(G).

Next we define some descriptional complexity measures. **Descriptional complexity measures** give information on the size and the structure of the grammar.

For a grammar G, **size measures** are the number of nonterminals and the number of productions of G, denoted by **Var**(G) and **Prod**(G), respectively.

In order to define **structural complexity** measures we need the next auxiliary notions:

Let $\triangleright$ be a binary relation on N such that for nonterminals X and Y we write $X \triangleright Y$ iff there is a production $X \to uYv$ in P, where $u,v \in (N \cup T)^*$. The reflexive and transitive closure of $\triangleright$ is denoted by $\triangleright^*$.

Two nonterminals X and Y are said to be structurally equivalent -denoted by $X \equiv Y$ - iff $X \triangleright^* Y$ and $Y \triangleright^* X$ hold. It can be seen immediately that $\equiv$ is an equivalence relation on N. Equivalence classes of N concerning $\equiv$ are said to be **grammatical levels** of G. The grammatical level containing the startsymbol is called the **initial level**.

For two grammatical levels Q_1 and Q_2 we write $Q_1 \rangle Q_2$ if there are nonterminals X and Y such that $X \in Q_1$, $Y \in Q_2$ and $X \triangleright Y$. The **digraph of grammatical levels** of G is defined as follows : its nodes are grammatical levels of G and there is an edge from node Q_1 to node Q_2 if $Q_1 \rangle Q_2$ holds.

Structural complexity measures are defined as follows; **Lev**(G) denotes the number of grammatical levels of G and **Hei**(G) denotes the length of the longest way, starting with the initial level, in the digraph of grammatical levels of G.

Formally,
$\mathbf{Hei}(G)= \max \{ \mathbf{Hei}(Q):Q$ is a grammatical level of G $\}$, where
$\mathbf{Hei}(Q)=1$ iff $S \in Q$ and $\mathbf{Hei}(Q_i)=1 + \max \{\mathbf{Hei}(Q_t) : Q_t \rangle Q_i \}$.

In the following we use the common notation K for **Var**, **Prod**, **Lev** and **Hei**.

We mean by the K-complexity of a language L, generated by grammars from a class **G** of grammars the following;

$$K_{\mathbf{G}}(L)=\min \{K(G) : L(G)=L, G \in \mathbf{G} \}.$$

The K-complexity of a class **L** of languages, generated by grammars from a class **G** of grammars -shortly the K-complexity of **L** with respect to **G** - is introduced as

$$K_{\mathbf{G}}(\mathbf{L})=\sup\{K_{\mathbf{G}}(L) : L \in \mathbf{L} \}.$$

Next we review the basic notions from grammar form theory. For detailed information see [W].

In the following all nonterminals and terminals are assumed to be elements of two fixed disjoint infinite sets, N and T , respectively.

A context-free grammar form and a general(strict) interpretation of it are defined as follows:

Let $G_i=(N_i,T_i,P_i,S_i)$, where i=1,2 be context-free grammars.We say that G_2 is a **general interpretation** (shortly a **g-interpretation**) of grammar form G_1 modulo μ, denoted by $G_2 \triangleleft_g G_1(\mu)$, where μ is a finite substitution on $(N_1 \cup T_1)^*$ if conditions (i)-(iv) obtain:

(i) $\mu(X) \subseteq N_2$ for all $X \in N_1$ and
if $X,Y \in N_1$ and $X \neq Y$ then $\mu(X) \cap \mu(Y) = \emptyset$;

(ii) $\mu(a) \subseteq T_2^*$ for all $a \in T_1$;

(iii) $P_2 \subseteq \mu(P_1) = \{u \to v: u \in \mu(r), v \in \mu(s), r \to s \in P_1\}$;

(iv) $S_2 \in \mu(S_1)$.

G_2 is said to be a **strict interpretation** of G_1 modulo μ, denoted by $G_2 \triangleleft_s G_1(\mu)$, (shortly an **s-interpretation**) if condition (ii) is modified in the following way:
$\mu(a) \subseteq T_2$ for all $a \in T_1$ and if $a,b \in T_1$ and $a \neq b$ then $\mu(a) \cap \mu(b) = \emptyset$.
The collection of x-interpretations of G_1, where $x \in \{g,s\}$ is said to be its **x-grammar family** and is denoted by $G_x(G_1)$.

The **x-grammatical family** of G_1 is defined as
$L_x(G_1) = \{L(G'): G' \in G_x(G_1)\}$.

By virtue of **reduction theorems** in grammar form theory completely reduced grammar forms have special importance (see [W]).

For a completely reduced grammar form G we define $G_{x,red}(G)$ and $L_{x,red}(G)$ as follows:

$G_{x,red}(G) = \{G': G' \in G_x(G)$ and G' is completely reduced$\}$;

$L_{x,red}(G) = \{L': L' = L(G'), G' \in G_{x,red}(G)\}$.

We note that if we consider a completely reduced grammar form G then $L_{s,red}(G) = L_s(G)$.

As the **empty word is relevant** from the point of view of **descriptional complexity**, therefore in the case of general interpretations we consider ε-free languages and ε-free grammars in the grammatical and the grammar family, respectively.

The degree of similarity in the grammar family can be characterized by the notion of a **(k,i)-bounded x-interpretation** of a grammar form : (see [CD])

Let $G_i = (N_i, T_i, P_i, S_i)$, $i=1,2$, be context-free grammars such that $G_2 \triangleleft_x G_1(\mu)$, where $x \in \{g,s\}$.
We say that G_2 is a **weak (k,i)-bounded x-interpretation** of G_1, where k and i are natural numbers if
(i) $card(\mu(X)) \leq k$ for all $X \in N_1$;
(ii) $card(\mu(a)) \leq i$ for all $a \in T_1$.
G_2 is said to be a **strong (k,i)-bounded x-interpretation** of G_1 if G_2 is a weak (k,i)-bounded x-interpretation of it and for all natural numbers l and m, where G_2 is a weak (l,m)-bounded x-interpretation of G_1, $k \leq l$ and $i \leq m$ hold. If condition (ii) is omitted then we speak of a **weak(strong) (k,∞)-bounded x-interpretation** of the grammar form.
The collection of strong (l,m)-bounded x-interpretations of G, where $l \leq k$ and $m \leq i$, is said to be the **(k,i)-bounded x-grammar family** of G and is denoted by $G_x^{(k,i)}(G)$.
Obviously, the **(k,∞)-bounded x-grammar family** of G, denoted by $G_x^{(k,\infty)}(G)$, is the collection of strong (j,∞)-bounded x-interpretations of G , where $j \leq k$.

The corresponding language collections, that is the **(k,i)-bounded x-grammatical family** and the **(k,∞)-bounded x-grammatical** family of G are defined as follows, respectively:
$L_x^{(k,i)}(G) = \{L' : L' = L(G'),\ G' \in G_x^{(k,i)}(G)\}$ and

$L_x^{(k,\infty)}(G) = \{L' : L' = L(G'),\ G' \in G_x^{(k,\infty)}(G)\}$.
These notions are extended for sets (collections) of languages in the usual way.

A grammar form is said to be nontrivial if it generates an infinite language.

A grammar form $G=(N,T,P,S)$ is said to be a **two-symbol form** if $N=\{S\}$ and $T=\{a\}$ hold.

Two-symbol forms have special importance in the theory of context-free languages as they produce the class of ε-free context-free languages by means of the **super-normal form theorem** as follows : (it can be found in [W])
Let $G=(\{S\},\{a\},P,S)$ be a two-symbol grammar form such that $L(G)=a^+$ and there is a production $S\text{->}w$ in P such that S occurs at least two times in w. Then $L_s(G)=L^{\varepsilon}(CF)$.
A grammar form F is said to be a **normal form grammar** if it satisfies the conditions of this theorem. A grammar G is said to be in **F-normal form** if it is a strict interpretation of F.

The most well-known types of normal forms of context-free grammars are Chomsky normal form grammars, Greibach normal form grammars and position restricted grammars (of type $t=(m_1,\ldots m_k,m_{k+1})$). For detailed informations and definitions see [K3].

For the connection with grammar form theory consider the following example:
for $G_{CH}=(\{S\},\{a\},\{S\text{->}SS,\ S\text{->}a\},S)$ $G_{s,red}(G_{CH})$ is equal to the class of completely reduced Chomsky normal form grammars and for $G_t=(\{S\},\{a\},\{S \text{->} a^{m_1}S\ldots a^{m_k}Sa^{m_{k+1}}, S\text{->}aS, S\text{->}a\},S)$ it holds that $G_{s,red}(G_t)$ is equal to the class of completely reduced position restricted grammars of type $t=(m_1,\ldots,m_k,m_{k+1})$.

We note that in [K3] those maximal subclasses of these normal form grammar classes are discussed which consist of completely reduced grammars.This consideration has a very simple reason: for example, if we assume the whole class of Chomsky normal form grammars, we can find for every context-free language L a grammar in Chomsky normal form generating L and having exactly one grammatical level.
It is a well-known fact that $L^{\varepsilon}(CF)=L(CH)=L(Gr)=L(t)$, where CH, Gr, t are those maximal subclasses of Chomsky normal form grammars, Greibach normal form grammars and position restricted grammars of type t, respectively, where all grammars are completely reduced.

In the following we consider only those normal form grammars (in the sense of W) which are completely reduced.

3. DESCRIPTIONAL COMPLEXITY MEASURES ON STRICT AND GENERAL GRAMMATICAL FAMILIES

In this section we consider those subclasses of context-free languages which are similarity classes, that is, they are general or strict grammatical families. We show that descriptional complexity measures **Lev**, **Var**, **Prod** are unbounded on every general(strict) grammatical family with respect to every general(strict) grammar family producing it. Moreover, in the case of strict grammatical families **Hei** is unbounded on the strict grammatical family, too. As $L^{\varepsilon}(CF)$ is a strict grammatical family, these results imply some well-known results from the area of descriptional complexity of context-free languages.

THEOREM 3.1.

Let G be a nontrivial completely reduced grammar form. Then **Lev**, **Var**, **Prod**, are unbounded on $L_{g,red}(G)$ with respect to $G_{g,red}(G)$.

PROOF

We first deal with complexity measure **Lev**. Let $G=(N,T,P,S)$. Assume first that $S \notin r(G)$. We shall construct an infinite sequence of languages $L^i \in L_{g,red}(G)$, where $i=1,2,\dots$, such that $Lev(L^i) < Lev(L^{i+1})$ for all $i=1,2,\dots$. Let $G^1=(N^1,T^1,P^1,S^1)$ be a completely reduced g-interpretation of G, defined by $G^1 \triangleleft_g G(\mu_1)$, such that for $L^1=L(G^1)$ $Lev(L^1)=Lev(G^1)$ holds. (It can be seen immediately that G^1 exists.) We construct L^2. Let $X \in r(G)$. Then there is a derivation d in G, where d: $S \overset{+}{\Rightarrow} uXv \overset{+}{\Rightarrow} urXsv \overset{+}{\Rightarrow} urwsv \in T^+$ holds and $rs \neq \varepsilon$. Denote by P_X the set of those productions of G which occur in this derivation. Let c be a new terminal such that $c \notin (T^1 \cup T \cup N^1 \cup N)$ and for every nonterminal $Y \in N$ let Y' be a new nonterminal such that $Y' \notin (T^1 \cup T \cup N^1 \cup N)$ and for all $Y,Z \in N$, where $Y \neq Z$, $Y' \neq Z'$ holds. Consider the following construction: for every $p \in P_X$, where $p = Y \to w_1Y_1w_2 \dots Y_nw_{n+1}$,

($n\geq 1$, $Y\in N$, $Y_i\in N, 1\leq i\leq n$, $w_j\in T^*$, $1\leq j\leq n+1$) let $p' = Y' \rightarrow c^{lg(w_1)} Y'_1 c^{lg(w_2)} \ldots Y'_n c^{lg(w_{n+1})}$, where a, Y' and Y'_i, $1\leq i\leq n$, are defined previously. Denote by P'_X the set of all productions obtained from P_X in this way. Let $G^2=(N^2,T^2,P^2,S')$ be a g-interpretation of G, defined by $G^2 \triangleleft_g G(\mu_2)$, where μ_2 is defined as follows: $\mu_2(Y)=(\mu_1(Y) \cup \{Y'\})$ for all $Y\in N$ and $\mu_2(a)=(\mu_1(a)\cup\{c\})$ for all $a\in T$. Let $N^2=\{Y':Y'\in\mu_2(Y), Y\in N\}$ and $T^2=\{a':a'\in\mu_2(a), a\in T\}$. Let $P^2=P^1\cup\{S'\rightarrow w: S^1\rightarrow w\in P^1\}\cup P'_X$. It is obvious, that for $L^2=L(G^2)$ $L^2=L^1\cup L^c$ holds, where L^c is an infinite context-free subset of c^+. (Evidently, L^1 and L^c are over disjoint alphabets.) We show that $\mathbf{Lev}(L^1)<\mathbf{Lev}(L^2)$ holds. Let $G''=(N'',T'',P'',S'')$ be a completely reduced grammar in $G_{g,red}(G)$ such that $L(G'')=L^2$ and $\mathbf{Lev}(G'')=\mathbf{Lev}(L^2)$. Denote by $N(L^1)$ the set of those nonterminals of G'' which are different from S'' and occur in at least one derivation of at least one word of L^1 and by $N(L^c)$ the set of those nonterminals which are different from S'' and are defined for L^c as defined for L^1. We prove that for arbitrary $Y\in N(L^1)$ and $Z\in N(L^c)$ it holds that Y and Z are in different grammatical levels of G''. Assume the contrary. As G'' is completely reduced, the following derivations exist:

d_1: $S''\overset{+}{\Rightarrow}uYv\overset{+}{\Rightarrow}uwv\in L^1$, where $Y\overset{+}{\Rightarrow}w$ and

d^2: $S''\overset{+}{\Rightarrow}uYv\overset{+}{\Rightarrow}urZsv\overset{+}{\Rightarrow}urtsv\overset{+}{\Rightarrow}w'$, where $r,s\in T''^+$, $t\in c^+$ and $Y\overset{+}{\Rightarrow}tZs$.

Then $w'\in L^2$ and w' is of form $w_1c^kw_2$, where $k\geq 1$ and w_1w_2 contains at least one letter from $alph(L^1)$. But this is a contradiction to that every word of L^2 consists of letters either of $alph(L^1)$ or of $alph(L^c)$. Thus, Y and Z are in different grammatical levels of G''. Using this type of considerations we can prove easily that elements of $N(L^1)$ and $N(L^c)$ cannot occur together in the same production of G''. Then $P''=P''^1\cup P''^c$, where P''^1 is the set of those productions in P'' in which all nonterminals are from $(N(L^1)\cup\{S''\})$ and P''^c is the set of those productions in P'' in which all nonterminals are from $(N(L^c)\cup\{S''\})$. Then $G''^1=((N(L^1)\cup\{S''\}),T^1,P''^1,S'')$ is a completely reduced g-interpretation of G and $L(G''^1)=L^1$. Then $\mathbf{Lev}(L^1)<\mathbf{Lev}(G''^1))$. Then $\mathbf{Lev}(L^2)=\mathbf{Lev}(G'')>\mathbf{Lev}(G''^1)+1$. Thus, $\mathbf{Lev}(L^2)>\mathbf{Lev}(L^1)$. Continuing these types of constructions of languages and applying the procedure for L^2 and so on, we obtain that if $S\notin r(G)$ then there is an infinite sequence of languages L^i, $i=1,2,\ldots$, such that $\mathbf{Lev}(L^i)<\mathbf{Lev}(L^{i+1})$ holds for all i. Thus, if $S\notin r(G)$ then Lev is unbounded on $L_{g,red}(G)$ with respect

to $G_{g,red}(G)$. Consider now the case when $S \in r(G)$. Then S can occur on the right-hand side of some element of P_X. Then we modify the construction in the following way: instead of G, as starting grammar we consider its g-interpretation $G'=(N',T,P',S)$, defined by $G' \triangleleft_g G(\mu')$ as follows: $\mu'(Z)=\{Z\}$ for all $Z \in (N \cup T)$, where $Z \neq S$ and $\mu'(S)=\{S,S'\}$, where $S' \notin (N \cup T)$. Let $P'=\mu(P)-\{p':p'$ contains S on its right-hand side$\}$. It is obvious that G' is completely reduced. Then we repeat the procedure written previously. As **Var**(L)$\geq$**Lev**(L) for every $L \in L_{g,red}(G)$, therefore we obtain immediately that **Var** is unbounded on $L_{g,red}(G)$ with respect to $G_{g,red}(G)$. Consider complexity measure **Prod**. Suppose that **Prod** is bounded on $L_{g,red}(G)$ with respect to $G_{g,red}(G)$. Then by virtue of the definition of a general interpretation, we obtain that **Var** is bounded on $L_{g,red}(G)$, which is a contradiction. Thus, **Prod** is unbounded on $L_{g,red}(G)$ with respect to $G_{g,red}(G)$.
Hence the result.

REMARK 3.1.
We consider completely reduced grammars for the same reason as it was mentioned in Section 2 (Preliminaries). Consider grammar form $G=(\{S\},\{a\},\{S\to SSS, S\to aS, S\to a\},S)$. It can be seen with simple considerations that for any language $L' \in L_s(G)$ there is a grammar G' in $G_s(G)$ that $L'=L(G')$ and **Lev**(G')=1 holds. Let $G\hat{}=(N\hat{},T\hat{},P\hat{},S\hat{}) \in G_s(G)$ such that $L(G\hat{})=L'$. Let $Y \notin N\hat{}$. Define P^1 as follows: for any $X \in N\hat{}$ let $p:X\to YXX$ and $q:Y\to XXY$ be elements of P^1. Then $G'=((N\hat{} \cup \{Y\}),T\hat{},P\hat{} \cup P^1,S\hat{})$ generates L' and **Lev**(G')=1.

We state an analogous result for strict grammatical families.

THEOREM 3.2.

let G be a nontrivial completely reduced grammar form. Then complexity measures **Hei**, **Lev**, **Var**, and **Prod** are unbounded on $L_s(G)$ with respect to $G_{s,red}(G)$.

PROOF

Let G=(N,T,P,S). We construct an infinite sequence of finite languages L^i, i=1,2,..., in $L_s(G)$ such that $\mathbf{Hei}(L^i)<\mathbf{Hei}(L^{i+1})$ holds for all i=1,2,..., with respect to $G_{s,red}(G)$. Consider the

following notation: for a $w \in L(G)$ and for a derivation tree t of w in G we denote by $d(t,w)$ the length of the longest branch of t. Let $m_1 \geq 2$ and let
$L^1 = \{w : w \in L(G), \min\{d(t,w) : t \text{ is a derivation tree of } w \text{ in } G\} \leq m_1\}$.
Let $lg(L^1) = \max\{lg(w) : w \in L^1\}$. As $L(G)$ is an ε-free infinite context-free language, therefore there is a word $w_2 \in L(G)$ such that $lg(w_2) > lg(L^1)$ holds. Then for $m_2 = \min\{d(t,w_2) : t$ is a derivation tree of w_2 in $G\}$ $m_2 > m_1$ holds. Let
$L^2 = \{w : w \in L(G), \min\{d(T,w) : t \text{ is a derivation tree of } w \text{ in } G\} \leq m_2\}$.
We define interpretations G^i generating finite languages L^i, for $i=1,2$, respectively. Consider those derivation trees t of every word in L^i which satisfy condition $d(t,w) \leq m_i$, $i=1,2$. Replace all nonterminal letters, occurring in these trees and different from the startsymbol, by different nonterminal letters such that every new nonterminal occurs in exactly one derivation tree exactly one times. Then collecting the productions obtained in this way (which were applied in the derivation trees), we obtain the production set of an s-interpretation G^i of G generating L^i, $i=1,2$, respectively. It is obvious, that $\mathbf{Hei}(G^2) = m_2 > m_1 > \mathbf{Hei}(L^1)$. Then applying this procedure for L^2 and so on, we obtain an infinite sequence of languages L^i, $i=1,2,\ldots$, such that $\mathbf{Hei}(L^i) < \mathbf{Hei}(L^{i+1})$ holds.
Thus, complexity measure **Hei** is unbounded on $L_s(G)$ with respect to $G_{s,red}(G)$. This result immediately implies that complexity measures **Lev**, **Var** and **Prod** are unbounded on $L_s(G)$ with respect to $G_{s,red}(G)$.
Hence the result.

COROLLARY 3.1.

Descriptional complexity measures **Lev**, **Hei**, **Var**, and **Prod** are unbounded on $L^{\varepsilon}(CF)$ with respect to $G_{s,red}(F)$, where F is a completely reduced normal form grammar.

The well-known results of Corollary 3.2. are special cases of Corollary 3.1.

COROLLARY 3.2

Descriptional complexity measures **Lev**, **Hei**, **Var**, **Prod** are unbounded

on $L^{\varepsilon}(CF)$ with respect to
(i) CH;
(ii) t , for arbitrary type $t=(m_1,\ldots,m_k,m_{k+1})$ of position restricted grammars.

REMARK 3.2.

Results of Corollary 3.2. can be found in [K3].

4. DESCRIPTIONAL COMPLEXITY MEASURES OF NORMAL FORMS OF CONTEXT-FREE GRAMMARS

In this section we show that the **Var**-complexity of an ε-free context-free language with respect to a class of completely reduced normal form grammars (in the sense of [W]) is equal to the degree of the boundness of the interpretation defining the **Var**-minimal grammar producing the language from the form grammar of this normal form class. We generalize some results of [K3] as we prove that for all natural numbers n and for all completely reduced normal form grammar classes F there is an ε-free context-free language L(n,K) such that the K-complexity of L(n,K) with respect to F is equal to n.

LEMMA 4.1.

Let F be a normal form grammar. Then

$$L_s^{(k,\infty)}(F)=F(k),$$

where F(k) denotes the family of languages generated by F-normal form grammars having at most k nonterminals.

The proof is a direct consequence of the corresponding definitions, therefore it is omitted.

REMARK 4.1.

The statement of Lemma 4.1. for the case of Chomsky normal form grammars was presented in [D].

Lemma 4.1. implies the next corollary.

COROLLARY 4.1.

(i) $CH(k)=L_s^{(k,\infty)}(G_{CH})$;

(ii) for every type $t=(m_1,\ldots,m_k,m_{k+1})$ of position restricted grammars
$t(k)=L_s^{(k,\infty)}(G_t)$,

where $CH(k)$ and $t(k)$ denote the classes of languages generated by Chomsky normal form grammars and position restricted grammars of type t having at most k nonterminals, respectively.

The next statement deals with the value of complexity measures on the strict grammatical family of a normal form grammar.

THEOREM 4.1.

For every positive integer n, for every normal form grammar F and for every complexity measure K there is a context-free language $L_F(n)$ such that

$$K(L_F(n))=n \quad \text{with respect to } G_{s,red}(F).$$

PROOF

The idea of the proof is based on the considerations of the idea of the proof of Theorem 3.2. Using the notation defined in that proof, we denote by d(t,w) the length of the longest branch of a derivation tree t of a word $w\in L(G)$ in G. Let
$L_F(n)=\{w:\min\{d(t,w):w\in L(G),t \text{ is a derivation tree of } w \text{ in } G\}\leq n\}$.
Let $k_n=\max\{lg(w):w\in L_F(n)\}$. Let $w_n\in L_F(n)$ such that $lg(w_n)=k_n$. Let $L_n(F)=\{w_n\}$. As F is a normal form grammar, we can see by simple considerations that the longest branch of any derivation tree of w_n is equal to n. We define an interpretation G^n of F which generates $L_F(n)$. We replace every letter S on the i-th level of

the derivation tree by S_i, $i=1,2,\ldots,n$ such that for $i\neq j$, $1\leq i,j\leq n$, $S_i\neq S_j$ holds. Denote the set of productions obtained in this way from the derivation tree by P^n. Then $G^n=(\{S_1,\ldots,S_n\},\{a\},P^n,S_1)$ is an s-interpretation of F and generates $L_F(n)=\{w_n\}$. By the construction we can see immediately that $K(L_F(n))=n$.
Hence the result.

The next statement of [K3] follows as a corollary from Theorem 4.1.

COROLLARY 4.2.

For every positive intger n and for every descriptional complexity measure K there are ε-free context-free languages $L_{CH}(n)$ and $L_t(n)$ such that

(i) $K(L_{CH}(n))=n$;

(ii) $K(L_t(n))=n$, where $t=(m_1,\ldots,m_k,m_{k+1})$ is an arbitrary type of position restricted grammars.

REFERENCES

[C] Csuhaj-Varjú,E. Some algebraic properties of k-bounded interpretations of grammar forms. Computational Linguistics and Computer Languages, XV,(John Benjamins B.V.), (1981),pp.76-113.

[CD] Csuhaj-Varjú,E.,Dassow,J. On bounded grammar forms, in preparation.

[D] Dassow,J. On bounded grammar forms,Manuscript,1984, TU Magdeburg.

[G1] Gruska,J. On a classification of context-free grammars, Kybernetika 3 (1967),22-29.

[G2] Gruska,J. Some classifications of context-free languages. Information and Control 14 (1969),152-179.

[G3] Gruska,J. Complexity and unambiguity of context-free languages. Information and Control 18 (1971),502-517.

[K1] Kelemenová,A. Grammatical levels of position restricted grammars, in: MFCS'81, (ed.by J.Gruska and M. Chytill), Lecture Notes in Computer Science 118, Springer-Verlag, (1981),347-359.

[K2] Kelemenová,A. Grammatical complexity of context-free languages and normal forms of context-free grammars, in: IMYCS'82, (ed.by P. Mikulecky),Bratislava ,(1982), 239-258.

[K3] Kelemenová,A. Complexity of normal form grammars, Theoretical Computer Science 28 (1984),288-314.

[S] Salomaa,A. Formal languages, Academic Press,1973.

[W] Wood,D. Grammar and L-forms:an introduction. Lecture Notes in Computer Science 91 ,Springer-Verlag, (1980)

BASIC IDEAS OF SELECTIVE SUBSTITUTION GRAMMARS

H.C.M. Kleijn
Department of Computer Science
University of Leiden
P.O. Box 9512
2300 RA Leiden
The Netherlands

INTRODUCTION

In this paper a general framework for the study of rewriting systems is discussed.
After some preliminaries the concept of a selective substitution grammar is presented and motivated in Section 2. In Section 3 we introduce s-grammars as instances of selective substitution grammars. This gives rise to a simple framework still general enough to characterize in a uniform way different features of rewriting systems. In the remainder of the paper we review the lines of research pursued until now. In Section 4 through 7 general approaches within the study of s-grammars are sketched. In Section 8 concrete classes of grammars are investigated in the framework of s-grammars, whereas in Section 9 a particular class of s-grammars, suited for an investigation of very basic properties of rewriting, is considered. Generalizations to two-dimensional and infinitary languages are briefly mentioned in Section 10. Finally, in Section 11, an extension to a general framework for the study of grammars and automata is discussed.

1. PRELIMINARIES

We assume the reader to be familiar with the basic concepts of formal language theory as, e.g., in the scope of Salomaa [27] and Rozenberg and Salomaa [25]. In addition the following notations and terminology are used.

Throughout the paper we assume that an infinite alphabet of

symbols is available: all symbols that will be used are elements of the infinite alphabet $\Lambda \cup \bar{\Lambda}$, where $\bar{\Lambda} = \{\bar{a} : a \in \Lambda\}$ and Λ and $\bar{\Lambda}$ are disjoint. A bar appearing above a symbol indicates that the original symbol is <u>activated</u>. Symbols without a bar are <u>non-activated</u>. Λ consists of non-activated symbols only. In the sequel all alphabets different from $\Lambda, \bar{\Lambda}$ or $\Lambda \cup \bar{\Lambda}$ are tacitly assumed to be finite.

For a word w, $|w|$ is its length and we denote the empty word by λ.

Let V and W be alphabets; $V, W \subseteq \Lambda \cup \bar{\Lambda}$.

(1). A total mapping h from V^* into non-empty subsets of W^* is a <u>substitution</u> (<u>from</u> V^* <u>into</u> W^*) if $h(\lambda) = \{\lambda\}$ and, for all $a \in V$ and $v \in V^*$, $h(av) = h(a)h(v)$. For $K \subseteq V^*$, $h(K) = \cup\{h(v) : v \in K\}$; h is a <u>finite substitution</u> if h(a) is finite for all $a \in V$.

(2). Let h be a finite substitution from V^* into W^*.

(2.1). h is a <u>finite-letter substitution</u> if $h(a) \subseteq W$, for all $a \in V$.

(2.2). h is a <u>homomorphism</u> if h(a) consists of one element for all $a \in V$; h is a <u>coding</u> if additionally $h(a) \subseteq W$ for all $a \in V$.

(2.3). h is a <u>weak identity</u> if it is a homomorphism, and for all $a \in V$, $h(a) = \{a\}$ or $h(a) = \{\lambda\}$.

The families of all substitutions, finite substitutions, finite-letter-substitutions, homomorphisms and codings from V^* into W^* are denoted by SUB(V,W), FSUB(V,W), FLSUB(V,W), HOM(V,W), and COD(V,W), respectively.

Let $h \in$ SUB(V,W). h is <u>non-erasing</u> if, for all $a \in V$, $\lambda \notin h(a)$. h is <u>disjoint</u> if, for all $v, w \in V^*$, such that $v \neq w$, $h(v) \cap h(w) = \emptyset$. If, for all $a \in V \cap \Lambda$, $h(a) \subseteq (W \cap \Lambda)^*$, and, for all $\bar{a} \in V \cap \bar{\Lambda}$, $h(\bar{a}) \subseteq (W \cap \bar{\Lambda})$, then h is called <u>bar-preserving</u>.

In the sequel we use a fixed coding *iden* $\in$ COD($\Lambda \cup \bar{\Lambda}, \Lambda$) to "remove bars". It is defined by *iden*(a) = *iden*($\bar{a}$) = {a}, for all $a \in \Lambda$. The restrictions of *iden* to subsets of $\Lambda \cup \bar{\Lambda}$ will also be denoted by *iden*.

A <u>context-free grammar</u> is specified as a 4-tuple (V,h,S,T), where V is its <u>total alphabet</u>, $T \subseteq V$ is its <u>terminal alphabet</u>, $S \in V-T$ its <u>axiom</u> (startsymbol) and $h \in$ FSUB(V-T,V) defines its <u>set of productions</u> in the following way: if $w \in h(a)$, for some $w \in V^*$ and $a \in V-T$, then (a,w) is a <u>production</u> and we write $(a,w) \in h$. The class of context-free grammars is denoted by CF.

An EOS <u>system</u> (see e.g., [19]) is, roughly speaking, a context-free grammar in which the rewriting of terminals is allowed. We specify it as a 4-tuple (V,h,S,T), where V and T are as for context-free grammars, $S \in V$, and $h \in$ FSUB(V,V) defines its set of productions. The class of EOS systems is denoted by EOS.

A context-free grammar (or EOS system) (V,h,S,T) is <u>propagating</u> if h is non-erasing. The class of propagating context-free grammars (EOS

systems) is denoted by Λ-CF (EPOS, respectively).
For a context-free grammar or EOS system G, the <u>direct derivation relation</u> $\Rightarrow_G$ is defined in the usual way. The <u>derivation relation</u> $\overset{*}{\Rightarrow}_G$ is its reflexive and transitive closure. The <u>language of</u> G, denoted by L(G), is defined by $L(G) = \{w \in T^* : S \overset{*}{\Rightarrow}_G w\}$.
The families of languages generated by context-free grammars and by EOS systems are denoted by L(CF) and L(EOS), respectively. Clearly L(CF) = L(EOS).

A context-free grammar (V,h,S,T) is <u>right-linear</u> if, for all $a \in V-T$, and for all $w \in h(a)$, $w \in T(V-T) \cup T \cup (V-T) \cup \{\Lambda\}$.
The class of (propagating) right-linear grammars is denoted by (Λ-)RLIN. The family of languages generated by right-linear grammars (i.e. the family of regular languages) is denoted by L(Reg).

The family of context-sensitive languages and the family of recursively enumerable languages are denoted by L(CS) and L(RE), respectively. We use ALL to denote the family of all languages.

2. SELECTIVE SUBSTITUTION GRAMMARS

Within formal language theory the notion of a rewriting system (or grammar) forms one of the most important tools in the study of formal languages. During the development of the grammatically oriented formal language theory numerous instances of rewriting systems have been defined, see e.g., Salomaa [27], and Dassow and Păun [3].
In 1977 Rozenberg proposed in [23] a unifying framework for rewriting systems. His aim was not to capture all existing rewriting systems in one general definition but rather to single out basic features of many kinds of rewriting systems and to define a general notion of a rewriting system based on these abstractions.
These basic features are the following:
- <u>Rewriting rules</u> or productions that describe the replacement (substitution) of single (occurrences of) letters.
- A <u>rewriting mechanism</u> that prescribes the use of productions in a word (selection) thus defining direct derivation steps.
- A <u>control</u> on the composition of sequences of direct derivation steps.
- A <u>language defining mechanism</u>.

Their abstractions when put together yield the notion of a <u>selective substitution grammar</u>.
We will abstain from giving the full formal definition of a selective

substitution grammar, but rather describe its components on an informal basis and relate them to the basic characteristics of rewriting systems as described above.

A selective substitution grammar is specified as a 7-tuple $G = (V,E,U,C,B,T,\psi)$.

$V \subseteq \mathcal{A}$ is the alphabet of G.

In G the rewriting of a single symbol is formalized using the notion of a based substitution. For $A \subseteq V$, an A-based substitution is a substitution $\delta \in SUB(V \cup \bar{A},V)$ such that $\delta(\bar{a}) \subseteq V^*$, for all $a \in A$ and $\delta(a) = \{a\}$, for all $a \in V$.

In a direct derivation step in G from a word $x \in V^*$, selected occurrences in x are replaced according to some based substitution in the following way. Given an A-based substitution $\delta \in SUB(V \cup \bar{A},V)$ and a selector (language) $K \subseteq (V \cup \bar{A})^*$, where $A \subseteq V$, one considers all words $y \in K$ that are equal to x upto bars, i.e. *iden*(y) = x. Each such y allows a rewriting in x of all and only those occurrences in x that have been activated (occur barred) in y.

The activated occurrences are replaced according to δ. Hence a word $x \in V^*$ directly derives a word $u \in V^*$, if and only if u is a result from an application of a selective substitution δ_K to x, where δ and K are as above. This means that $u \in \delta_K(x)$, where

$\delta_K(x) = \cup\{\delta(y) : y \in K \text{ and } iden(y) = x\}$.

In general G has several selective substitutions which are specified in U, the set of substitution blocks of G. $U = \{\varphi_e : e \in E\}$ where E is the set of labels of G and each φ_e is a selective substitution with an underlying A_e-based substitution δ^e and a selector $K_e \subseteq (V \cup \bar{A}_e)^*$, for some $A_e \subseteq V$.

Now sequences of direct derivation steps, each using a selective substitution φ_e as described above, are composed according to the control set C of G, where $C \subseteq E^*$. For $c = e_1 \ldots e_n$, where $n \geq 1$ and $e_i \in E$, for $1 \leq i \leq n$, φ_c denotes the composition $\varphi_{e_n} \circ \ldots \circ \varphi_{e_1}$; $\varphi_\Lambda(x) = \{x\}$, for all $x \in V^*$. For $x,u \in V^*$, x derives u according to some $c \in E^*$, denoted by $x \Rightarrow^c u$, if $u \in \varphi_c(x)$. In G only derivations $x \Rightarrow^c u$ such that $c \in C$ are allowed.

The language of G, L(G) is obtained by considering all words that can be derived from words in $B \subseteq V^*$, the set of axioms (startwords) of G, and then applying to them a (partial) mapping ψ (the filter of G) from V^* into T^*, where T is the terminal alphabet of G.

Hence $L(G) = \{w \in T^* :$ there exist a word $x \in B$ and a word $u \in V^*$ such that $x \Rightarrow^c u$, for some $c \in C$, and $\psi(u) = w\}$.

In [23] Rozenberg demonstrates the flexibility of the framework of selective subsitution grammars by showing how a variety of classes of grammars fits into it. Two of these examples are provided here.

Example 2.1. Let $G = (V,E,U,C,B,T,\psi)$ be a selective substitution grammar, where

(1). $B = \{S\}$, with $S \in V-T$, $E = \{e\}$, $C = E^*$, $T \subseteq V$, ψ is a partial identity mapping defined on T only, $U = \{\varphi_e\}$, with $\varphi_e = \delta_K$, $K = V^*(\overline{V-T})V^*$ and $\delta \in FSUB(V \cup (\overline{V-T}),V)$.

Then G is interpreted as a context-free grammar.

(2). $B = \{w\}$, with $w \in V^*$, $C = E^*$, $T \subseteq V$, ψ is a partial identity mapping defined on T only, each φ_e in U, for $e \in E$, is of the form δ_K^e with $K = \overline{V}^*$ and $\delta^e \in FSUB(V \cup \overline{V},V)$.

Then G is interpreted as an ETOL system (see Rozenberg and Salomaa [25]). Note that if U contains only one substitution block, then we are dealing with an EOL system. □

3. s-GRAMMARS

As the notion of a selective substitution grammar provides a framework for a general theory of rewriting systems it is rather involved. In order to investigate various properties of rewriting systems it is useful to restrict this framework to a more concrete and simpler one, in which the features one is interested in are high-lighted.

The most striking aspect of selective substitution grammars is the explicit way (by selectors) of selecting the occurrences to be rewritten which is more implicit in most classes of grammars. This motivated Rozenberg and Wood in [26] to use context-free grammars with selection as special instances of selective substitution grammars in order to gain more understanding of the role of selection. In later research also the possiblility of rewriting terminals is taken into account.

This has led to the introduction of s-grammars which provide a simple framework still general enough for a unified approach to the study of rewriting systems. (See Kleijn [17]). Here we introduce the notion of an s-grammar as a restricted version of a selective substitution grammar with one startletter, one substitution block, the standard filter, and implicit control.

Let $G = (V,E,U,C,B,T,\psi)$ be a selective substitution grammar and let $A \subseteq V$ be a fixed set of symbols, the active symbols of G.

Furthermore, let $B = \{S\}$, with $S \in A$, $E = \{e\}$, $C = E^*$, $T \subseteq V$, ψ is a partial identity mapping defined on T only, $U = \{\varphi_e\}$ with $\varphi_e = \delta_K$, for some $K \subseteq (V \cup \bar{A})^*$ and $\delta \in FSUB(V \cup \bar{A}, V)$.
Now G can be specified in the form (V,h,S,T,K), where $h \in FSUB(A,V)$ is defined by $h(a) = \delta(\bar{a})$, for all $a \in A$.
(V,h,S,T) is called the <u>base of</u> G and denoted by *base*(G), and K is called the <u>selector</u> of G and denoted by *sel*(G). We use A(G) to denote the <u>set of active symbols of</u> G.
Note that, for A(G) = V-T, *base*(G) is the specification of a context-free grammar and, for A(G) = V, it is the specification of an EOS system. In the former case we refer to G as a <u>CF-based s-grammar</u> and in the latter case we refer to it as an <u>EOS-based s-grammar</u>. If G is an X-based s-grammar, with $X \in \{CF, EOS\}$, we may also refer to it as an <u>s-grammar</u>.
The rewriting process in an s-grammar G = (V,h,S,T,K) can easily be described: $x \in V^*$ can be rewritten if and only if K contains a word y that is equal to x upto bars. The rewriting of x is now performed by applying productions from h to exactly those occurrences in x that correspond to barred (activated) occurrences in the chosen selector word y. All other occurrences remain untouched. The language of the grammar is the set of all words over the terminal alphabet T of G that can be derived from its axiom S by iterating this procedure. Formally we have the following definitions.
Let G = (V,h,S,T,K) be an s-grammar.
For $x, u \in V^*$, x <u>directly derives</u> u (<u>in</u> G) if there exists a word $y \in K$, such that *iden*(y) = x, and if $y = a_1 \ldots a_n$, for $a_i \in V \cup \overline{A(G)}$, $1 \le i \le n$, then $u = w_1 \ldots w_n$ where, for $1 \le i \le n$, $w_i = a_i$ if $a_i \in V$ and $w_i \in h(iden(a_i))$ if $a_i \in \overline{A(G)}$. Let $\Rightarrow_G$ denote the direct derivation relation in G; then $\overset{*}{\Rightarrow}_G$ is its reflexive and transitive closure.
The <u>language of</u> G, denoted as L(G), is now defined by
$L(G) = \{w \in T^* : S \overset{*}{\Rightarrow}_G w\}$.

Example 3.1. Let G = (V,h,S,T,K) be an s-grammar.
(1). $K = V^* \overline{A(G)} V^*$.
Then L(G) = L(*base*(G)), since the rewriting procedure described by K corresponds to the rewriting in the underlying CF-grammar (A(G) = V-T) or EOS-system (A(G) = V).
(2). $K = \bigcup_{i=1}^{n} \bar{V}_i^*$, with $V_i \subseteq A(G)$, for $1 \le i \le n$.
Then G corresponds to an ETOL system with (partial) tables $h_1, \ldots, h_n$ where, for $1 \le i \le n$, $h_i(a) = h(a)$, for $a \in V_i$, and $h_i(a)$ is not defined otherwise. □

The following important observations are immediate consequences of the definitions.

Theorem 3.1. Let G be an s-grammar.
(1). $L(G) \subseteq L(\textit{base}(G))$.
(2). If $V^*\overline{A(G)}V^* \subseteq \textit{sel}(G)$, where V is the alphabet of G, then $L(G) = L(\textit{base}(G))$. □

A selector is a language over (a finite subset of) $A \cup \bar{A}$. Any family of languages over $A \cup \bar{A}$ will be called a <u>family of selectors</u>. One obtains different classes of s-grammars by varying the families of selectors and by varying the classes of bases. Let X be a class of context-free grammars or a class of EOS systems and let K be a family of selectors. Then $(X,K) = \{G : G$ is an s-grammar with $\textit{base}(G) \in X$ and $\textit{sel}(G) \in K\}$ and $L(X,K) = \{L(G) : G \in (X,K)\}$.

In the theory of s-grammars research is focussed on the interrelationships between classes of selectors, classes of bases and families of languages generated by s-grammars with certain bases and selectors. Before we describe the ideas underlying the research until now and some of the results obtained so far, we first discuss the relationship between CF-based s-grammars and EOS-based s-grammars in order to facilitate our later considerations.
As we have seen $L(CF) = L(EOS)$ and for many questions in formal language theory it does not matter whether or not it is allowed to rewrite terminals. In a general theory of rewriting systems, however, this difference may become important. In the case of s-grammars it is obvious that every CF-based s-grammar can be viewed as an EOS-based s-grammar which has only, say, identity productions for its terminal symbols.

Theorem 3.2. For every selector K, $L(CF,\{K\}) \subseteq L(EOS,\{K\})$. □

On the other hand, in general an EOS-based s-grammar cannot directly be interpreted as a CF-based s-grammar without changing its selector. Since in a CF-based s-grammar terminal symbols cannot be activated (occur barred in the selector), also the selector of an EOS-based s-grammar has to be transformed in some way in order to arrive at a CF-based s-grammar. If a certain family K of selectors is closed under such a transformation, then $L(CF,K) = L(EOS,K)$. We discuss briefly a transformation from EOS-based s-grammars to CF-based s-grammars preserving equivalence and the family of selectors involved, if that is closed under a certain operation.

Let $G = (V,h,S,T,K)$ be an EOS-based s-grammar. Let $T' = \{a' : a \in T\}$ and let $f \in FLSUB(V \cup \overline{V}, V \cup T' \cup \overline{(V-T)} \cup \overline{T}')$ be defined by $f(a) = \{a\}$, for $a \in (V-T) \cup \overline{(V-T)}$, $f(a) = \{a,a'\}$, for $a \in T$, and $f(\overline{a}) = \{\overline{a}'\}$, for $a \in T$. Define the finite substitution $g \in FSUB((V-T) \cup T', V \cup T')$ by $g(a) = f(h(a))$, for $a \in V-T$, and $g(a') = f(h(a))$, for $a \in T$. Let $Z = S$, if $S \in V-T$, and let $Z = S'$, if $S \in T$. Then $H = (V \cup T',g,Z,T,f(K))$ is a CF-based s-grammar and $L(H) = L(G)$.
The transformation f applied to K is a disjoint and bar-preserving finite-letter-substitution. If K is a family of selectors that is closed under disjoint and bar-preserving finite-letter-substitutions, then we say that K is dbpfls. Hence we have the following result.

Theorem 3.3. If K is a dbpfls family of selectors, then $L(CF,K) = L(EOS,K)$. □

4. FAMILIES OF SELECTORS

A natural first step in the investigation of s-grammars is to investigate how "big" a family of selectors should be in order to define a "reasonable" family of languages. (This topic is addressed in Rozenberg and Wood [26].) It turns out that when no restrictions are imposed on the selectors any language can be generated by an s-grammar.

Example 4.1. Let $T \subseteq A$ and let $L \subseteq T^*$ be an arbitrary language. The CF-based s-grammar $G = (V,h,S,T,K)$ is defined by $V = \{S,Z\} \cup T$; $h(S) = \{aS : a \in T\} \cup \{Z\}$ and $h(Z) = \{\Lambda\}$; $K = T^*\overline{S} \cup L\overline{Z}$.
Then $L(G) = L$. □

Hence we have

Theorem 4.1. $L(RLIN,ALL) = ALL$. □

Corollary 4.1. $L(CF,ALL) = L(EOS,ALL) = ALL$. □

Example 4.1. also implies that for $K \in \{L(RE), L(CS), L(CF), L(Reg)\}$, $L(RLIN,K) \supseteq K$. Hence much of the generative capacity of s-grammars stems from the possibility of encoding the desired language in the selector. It is, however, desirable to define languages using objects that are less complicated than these languages themselves. In case of $\mathcal{L}(\mathrm{RE})$ it turns out to be sufficient to consider only regular selectors.

Theorem 4.2. $\mathcal{L}(\mathrm{CF},\mathcal{L}(\mathrm{Reg})) = \mathcal{L}(\mathrm{CF},\mathcal{L}(\mathrm{CF})) = \mathcal{L}(\mathrm{CF},\mathcal{L}(\mathrm{CS})) = \mathcal{L}(\mathrm{CF},\mathcal{L}(\mathrm{RE})) = \mathcal{L}(\mathrm{RE})$. □

Since $\mathcal{L}(\mathrm{Reg})$, $\mathcal{L}(\mathrm{CF})$, $\mathcal{L}(\mathrm{CS})$, and $\mathcal{L}(\mathrm{RE})$ are dbpfls a similar result holds for EOS-based s-grammars. When we impose additional restrictions on the bases the situation changes:

Theorem 4.3. $\mathcal{L}(\Lambda\text{-RLIN},\mathcal{L}(\mathrm{RE})) = \mathcal{L}(\Lambda\text{-CF},\mathcal{L}(\mathrm{RE})) = \mathcal{L}(\mathrm{RE})$.
$\mathcal{L}(\Lambda\text{-CF},\mathcal{L}(\mathrm{Reg})) = \mathcal{L}(\Lambda\text{-CF},\mathcal{L}(\mathrm{CF})) = \mathcal{L}(\Lambda\text{-CF},\mathcal{L}(\mathrm{CS})) = \mathcal{L}(\mathrm{CS})$.
$\mathcal{L}(\Lambda\text{-RLIN},\mathcal{L}(\mathrm{Reg})) \subset \mathcal{L}(\Lambda\text{-RLIN},\mathcal{L}(\mathrm{CF})) \subset \mathcal{L}(\Lambda\text{-RLIN},\mathcal{L}(\mathrm{CS})) = \mathcal{L}(\mathrm{CS})$. □

For more detailed considerations we refer to Rozenberg and Wood [26].

5. STRUCTURAL RESTRICTIONS ON SELECTORS

As we have seen even with rather restricted families of selectors, s-grammars can still generate complicated families of languages. But some restrictions have more influence on the language generating power than others. From Example 3.1. it follows that with selectors of the form $V^*\overline{V}V^*$ all and only context-free languages are generated whereas s-grammars with selectors of the form $\overline{V}^*$ generate the EOL languages. Such considerations lead to the question what features of selectors are responsible for the language generating power of s-grammars.
Intuitively the language generating power of a selector stems from the possibilities it has to use information from the context in the rewriting process and the possibility of blocking a derivation (by not providing a matching selector word for the current sentential form) if something goes wrong. In Rozenberg and Wood [26] some aspects of the above features are formalized and then investigated for their effects on the language generating power. In Kleijn and Rozenberg [19] this study is continued in more detail. Using context-free grammars as an example of grammars where context-information does not influence the rewriting process, and where no essential derivation-blocking possibilities are present, various "context-free" restrictions are imposed on the selectors of s-grammars. All combinations of these restrictions have been investigated. Some combinations of restrictions

yield characterizations of the context-free languages, for some combinations lower- and upperbounds on the language generating power of the resulting s-grammars can be given, whereas there are also combinations which do not restrict the language generating power. Roughly four types of restrictions are distinguished in [19] and formalized as conditions to be satisfied by s-grammars.
- Bar-freeness, which forbids to program the choice of particular places in a string to be rewritten.
- Interspersion, which forbids to test on the immediate neighbourhood of letters.
- Symbol-freeness, which forbids to distinguish between symbols that should or should not appear at particular places in a word.
- Universality, which requires that every word containing an active symbol can be rewritten.

Here we only give formal definitions for symbol-freeness (which is also investigated in Section 9) and universality.

Let $G = (V,h,S,T,K)$ be an s-grammar.
G is symbol-free if, for every $w_1,w_2 \in V \cup \overline{A(G)}^*$ and for every $a \in A(G)$ and $b \in V$, whenever, $w_1\bar{a}w_2 \in K$, then $w_1\overline{A(G)}w_2 \subseteq K$, and whenever $w_1bw_2 \in K$, then $w_1Vw_2 \subseteq K$.
G is universal if, for every $w \in V^*A(G)V^*$, there exists a word $v \in K$, such that $v \neq w$ and *iden*$(v) = w$.
Note that the s-grammar $G = (V,h,S,T,V^*\overline{A(G)}V^*)$ is both symbol-free and universal. Hence the class of context-free languages constitutes a lowerbound on the generative power of the symbol-free and universal s-grammars. The s-grammar $G = (V,h,S,T,\overline{A(G)}^*)$ is symbol-free. If G is CF-based it is not universal. In case G is EOS-based, however, it is universal. Hence all EOL languages can be generated by symbol-free and universal EOS-based s-grammars. The next result shows that these s-grammars can even generate languages with arbitrarily complicated length sets.

Theorem 5.1. Let $R \subseteq \mathbb{N}$.
There exists a symbol-free and universal EOS-based s-grammar G such that $R = \{ |w| : w \in L(G) \}$. □

For the case of CF-based s-grammars one can only prove the following theorem.

Theorem 5.2. Let $R \subseteq \mathbb{N}$.
There exists a symbol-free CF-based s-grammar G such that $R = \{ |w| : w \in L(G) \}$. □

This difference is explained by the following result.

Theorem 5.3. (1). All languages can be generated by universal EOS-based s-grammars.
(2). A language is context-free if and only if it can be generated by a universal CF-based s-grammar. □

Hence in case the rewriting of terminals is not allowed, universality provides a characterization of the context-free languages. In Kleijn and Rozenberg [19] the difference between CF-based s-grammars and EOS-based s-grammars under all combinations of restrictions is further investigated. Here we stress that transformations between the two types of s-grammars as described in Section 3 of this paper are not guaranteed to preserve the restrictions imposed on s-grammars, e.g., a universal CF-based s-grammar cannot directly be interpreted as a universal EOS-based s-grammar.

As regards the bases we can add the following remarks. In Kleijn and Rozenberg [19] only propagating bases (i.e. from Λ-CF and EPOS) are considered. This, however, does not affect the results as we have stated them here. In Gonczarowski et al. [14] for some combinations of restrictions it is shown that they do not affect the language generating power even in the case that the bases satisfy additional requirements. (See also Section 7.)

6. PROPERTIES OF GENERATED LANGUAGES

Until now we have concentrated on the influence of the properties of the selector of an s-grammar on the language generated by the s-grammar. Another approach is to consider certain properties of (families of) languages and to try to find conditions on (families of) selectors guaranteeing those desired properties for the (families of) languages generated by the corresponding s-grammars. In Gonczarowski et al. [12,13] and in Chapter 5 of Kleijn [17] this line of research is pursued for closure properties. In [12,13] a wide range of language theoretical operations is considered. Then, for each of those operations, conditions on selector families are formulated which guarantee that the families of languages generated by the corresponding s-grammars are closed under this operation. A number of these general results is applied to prove that some specific families of languages are closed under certain operations. This demonstrates once more the usefulness of having a general theory of rewriting systems. The first part of Chapter 5 of [17] is based on the research presented in [12,13] and focusses on AFL closure properties.

A family of languages is called an <u>abstract family of languages</u> (an AFL for short), if it contains a non-empty language and is closed under each of the following operations: union, Kleene cross, non-erasing homomorphism, inverse homomorphism, and intersection with regular languages. An AFL is <u>full</u> if it is closed under arbitrary homomorphism.

For each of the above properties a set of conditions on families of selectors is presented guaranteeing that the families of languages generated by the corresponding classes of s-grammars have this property. The combination of conditions yields the following result.

Theorem 6.1. Let K be a dbpfls family of selectors that satisfies all of the following conditions.

(1). There exists a $K \in K$, such that $K \cap \bar{A} \neq \emptyset$.

(2). K is closed under union.

(3). K is closed under union with languages of the form $\bar{W}^*$ with $W \subseteq A$.

(4). K is closed under concatenation with languages of the form W^* with $W \subseteq A$.

Then $L(EOS,K) = L(CF,K)$ is a full AFL. □

7. BASES

Having investigated the relationship between families of selectors and families of languages generated by s-grammars using these selectors, we now turn to considerations explicitly involving the bases of s-grammars. Some attention to the role of the bases has already been given in previous sections. In particular s-grammars with bases from CF and s-grammars with bases from EOS have been compared and possibilities of performing transformations without affecting the families of selectors or the language generating power have been considered. In fact the topic of grammatical transformations (to a certain "normal form") is a traditional one in formal language theory. In Gonczarowski et al. [14] and in the second part of Chapter 5 of Kleijn [17] which is based on [14], "standard" grammatical transformations are considered in the framework of s-grammars (as suggested in [26]). Whether or not a transformation can be performed within a given class of s-grammars depends on the family of selectors involved. This leads to the formulation of conditions on selector families. The results obtained are applied to specific classes of s-grammars. Here we present a result from [17].

An s-grammar (V,h,S,T,K) is <u>binary</u> (has a <u>binary base</u>), if, for all $a \in A(G)$ and $w \in V^*$, $w \in h(a)$ implies $|w| \leq 2$.
To perform a more or less standard transformation to binary bases within a certain class of s-grammars, we use the following notion.
Let $V \subseteq A \cup \bar{A}$ and let $t \in A$ be such that $\{t,\bar{t}\} \cap V = \emptyset$. A substitution $g \in SUB(V, V \cup \{t,\bar{t}\})$ such that, for $a \in V \cap A$, $g(a) = t^* a t^*$ and, for $\bar{a} \in V \cap \bar{A}$, $g(\bar{a}) = \bar{t}^* \overline{at}^*$ is called an <u>r-substitution</u> (<u>for</u> V <u>and</u> t).

Theorem 7.1. Let K be a dbpfls family of selectors that is closed under union and r-substitution. Then, for every $G \in (EOS, K)$ there exists an equivalent binary $G' \in (EOS, K)$. □

At this point one should notice the difference between the existence of a normal form for bases and the possibility of changing bases without leaving a certain family of selectors. Note that by Example 4.1, for every language L, a binary s-grammar exists that generates L. In Gonczarowski et al. [14] it is shown that certain standard restrictions as, e.g., chain-freeness, imposed on the bases (even when combined with additional restrictions on the selectors as discussed in Section 5) do not affect the language generating power of the <u>whole</u> class of s-grammars. From Example 4.1 an even stronger normal form for bases follows: one <u>fixed</u> base suffices to generate all languages (over a fixed terminal alphabet). This leads to the following notions, which are introduced and discussed in Rozenberg and Wood [26].

. Let Y be a class of context-free grammars or EOS systems and let K be a family of selectors. Let $T \subseteq A$.
$G \in Y$ is said to be K-<u>universal</u> <u>for</u> Y <u>modulo</u> T if
$L(\{G\},K)=\{L \subseteq T^* : L \in L(Y,K)\}$.
$K \in K$ is said to be Y-<u>universal</u> <u>for</u> K <u>modulo</u> T if
$L(Y,\{K\}) = \{L \subseteq T^* : L \in L(Y,K)\}$.
(The interested reader may also look up Gonczarowski et al. [14] for the related notion of s-generator.)
Now one can investigate what conditions on a selector family K guarantee the existence of a K-universal base. From Example 4.1. it follows that for every alphabet $T \subseteq A$ there exists a context-free grammar (EOS system) that is K-universal for CF (EOS) modulo T, where K is any family closed under union with regular languages and

"endmarking". This can be applied to specific families of selectors as e.g., ALL, $\mathcal{L}$(RE), $\mathcal{L}$(CS), $\mathcal{L}$(CF), and $\mathcal{L}$(Reg). The next result (from Rozenberg and Wood [26]) is proved using transformations to a fixed base.

Theorem 7.2. Let K be a family of selectors, that is closed under union and finite substitutions. Let $T \subseteq A$. There exists a context-free grammar that is K-universal for CF modulo T. □

For the grammar-universality of families of selectors we do not present results as it is a more restricted notion than the selector-universality of bases. A fixed selector prohibits the possibility of encoding directly the languages to be generated and moreover it establishes an upperbound on the number of non-terminals that can be used actively in the base.

8. SPECIFIC SELECTORS

In this section we present an example of the study of concrete "rewriting modes" prescribed by specific families of selectors. Such research is presented in Ehrenfeucht et al. [11], Kleijn and Rozenberg [20] and continued in Kleijn and Rozenberg [21], Ehrenfeucht et al. [10], and Subramanian [30].
Sequential and parallel rewriting modes are investigated and compared in the framework of s-grammars, together with a new "in-between" continuous way of rewriting. Using context-free grammars (selectors of the form $V^*(\overline{V-T})V^*$) and EOL systems (selectors of the form $\overline{V}^*$) as extreme examples of sequential and parallel rewriting three classes of s-grammars are introduced. Sequential grammars (rewriting only one occurrence in a derivation step), parallel grammars (rewriting all occurrences in a derivation step), and continuous grammars (rewriting a continuous segment in a derivation step).

Let $n \geq 1$.
The family of n-sequential selectors, denoted by nS, is defined by
$nS = \{\bigcup_{i=1}^{n} X_i^*\overline{Y}_iZ_i^* : X_i,Y_i,Z_i \subseteq A, \text{ for } 1 \leq i \leq n\}$.
The family of n-parallel selectors, denoted by nL, is defined by
$nL = \{\bigcup_{i=1}^{n} \overline{Y}_i^* : Y_i \subseteq A, \text{ for } 1 \leq i \leq n\}$.
The family of n-continuous selectors, denoted by nC, is defined by
$nC = \{\bigcup_{i=1}^{n} X_i^*\overline{Y}_i^+Z_i^* : X_i,Y_i,Z_i \subseteq A, \text{ for } 1 \leq i \leq n\}$.

An s-grammar G is called <u>sequential</u> (<u>parallel</u>, <u>continuous</u>) if *sel*(G) ∈ nS (nL,nC), for some n ≥ 1.
Note that nS, nC, and nL are dbpfls families of selectors. Hence by Theorem 3.3, *L*(EOS,*K*) = *L*(CF,*K*), for *K* ∈ {nS,nC,nL}.
Much emphasis has been given to the investigation of the language generating power of these classes of s-grammars both in relation to one another and in relation to known classes (see [10], [11], [20]). Not all questions have been solved yet. In [12,13] and [17] an application of the results on closure properties (see Section 6) yields that the family of languages generated by continuous grammars is an AFL. This has also independently and directly been proved in [30]. In [20] and [21] also the role of erasing productions is considered and combinations of sequential, continuous and parallel selectors are investigated. The sequential, continuous and parallel modes of rewriting are investigated further (in [20]) by subjecting them to certain fundamental restrictions as context-symmetry and selection determinism. This brings to light essential differences between sequential, continuous and parallel grammars and yields new characterizations for several known classes of languages.

9. PATTERN GRAMMARS

Within the framework of s-grammars it is possible to consider special classes of s-grammars which in their turn are sufficiently "broad" to allow a unified approach to the basics of rewriting processes. The class of pattern grammars (introduced in Kleijn and Rozenberg [19]) forms such a concrete framework. A pattern grammar is actually a symbol-free s-grammar (see Section 5). In such an s-grammar the symbols occurring in the selector are not relevant. The only thing that matters is whether or not they occur activated (barred). Hence the selector controls the rewriting only by prescribing "rewriting patterns" which can be viewed as consisting of two symbols: 1 for "rewrite" and 0 for "do not rewrite". Varying the rewriting patterns leads to very different rewriting systems. For instance, a context-free grammar uses rewriting patterns from 0^*10^* (i.e. rewrite one occurrence) and an EOL system uses patterns from 1^* (i.e. rewrite all occurrences).
In the remainder of this section 0 and 1 are distinguished symbols.

A <u>pattern grammar</u> is a construct G = (V,h,S,T,K) where

base(G)=(V,h,S,T) is a context-free grammar or an EOS system and *sel*(G) = K $\subseteq$ $\{0,1\}^*$.
Let $s_{V,A(G)} \in FSUB(\{0,1\}, V \cup \overline{A(G)})$ be defined by $s_{V,A(G)}(0) = V$ and $s_{V,A(G)}(1) = A(G)$. Then $s(G) = (V,h,S,T,s_{V,A(G)}(K))$ is the symbol-free s-grammar corresponding to G. The direct derivation relation and derivation relation in G are inherited from s(G) and L(G) = L(s(G)). Note that a symbol-free s-grammar H = (V,h,S,T,K) corresponds to the pattern grammar $s^{-1}(H) = (V,h,S,T,s^{-1}_{V,A(H)}(H))$ and $ss^{-1}(H) = H$. Hence symbol-free s-grammars and pattern grammars specify the same objects. However, since the selectors of pattern grammars do not involve the names of symbols they facilitate a general approach: One language $K \subseteq \{0,1\}^*$ determines a family of selectors $\{s_{V,A}(K) : A \subseteq V \subseteq A\}$. Any language over {0,1} will be called a pattern selector. Using observations similar to those in Section 3, it can easily be seen that, for pattern grammars - even in the case of one fixed pattern selector - the difference between EOS bases and CF bases can be discarded. For a family *K* of pattern selectors, *L*(p*K*) = {L(G) : G is a pattern grammar with *sel*(G) $\in$ *K*}. Let Pat denote the family of all pattern selectors and let RegPat denote the family of all regular pattern selectors. From Theorem 5.2. it follows that *L*(pPat) contains arbitrarily complicated languages. In Kleijn and Rozenberg [19] and [22] the generative power of regular pattern grammars (pattern grammars with a regular selector) is investigated. This leads to the following results.

Theorem 9.1. (1). *L*(pRegPat) $\subseteq$ *L*(RE).
(2). For every L $\in$ *L*(RE), $L¢^5$ $\in$ *L*(pRegPat), where ¢ is a new symbol.
(3). For every L $\in$ *L*(RE), there exists a weak identity g and a propagating regular pattern grammar G such that L = g(L(G)). □

Hence even the simple class of regular pattern grammars generates "almost" the recursively enumerable languages. This generative power seems to stem from the "counting" ability of regular pattern selectors. In order to destroy this ability two additional restrictions are considered in [22].
$K \subseteq \{0,1\}^*$ is commutative if, for all $x,y \in \{0,1\}^*$, x01y $\in$ K if and only if x10y $\in$ K.
$K \subseteq \{0,1\}^*$ is prefix closed if, for all $x,y \in \{0,1\}^*$, xy $\in$ K implies that x$\in$K.
The family of commutative and prefix closed regular patterns is denoted by CPRegPat.

Theorem 9.2. *L*(EOL) $\subset$ *L*(pCPRegPat) $\subset$ *L*(CS). □

Interesting examples of rewriting patters are $0^*1^k0^*$ and $0^*(10^*)^k$, $k \geq 1$, which determine "context-free" grammars in which in every derivation step k (adjacent or scattered) symbols are rewritten in parallel. (The rewriting of the axiom is "free".) It is easy to see that, for $k \geq 2$, the patterns $0^*(10^*)^k$ give rise to non context-free languages, as, e.g. $\{a_1^n \dots a_k^n : n \geq 1\}$. For the adjacent case it remained for some time an open problem whether or not $L(p\{0^*110^*\})$ contains non context-free languages (see [18]). This problem has recently been solved by Dahlhaus and Gaifman [2], who showed that $L(p\{0^*110^*\})$ contains non EOL languages.

Theorem 9.3. $L(CF) \subset L(p\{0^*110^*\})$. □

In Gonczarowski and Shamir [15] and Gonczarowski and Warmuth [16] parsing algorithms are developed and the complexities of the membership problems are investigated for families $L(p\{0^*1^k0^*\})$ and $L(p\{0^*(10^*)^k\})$, $k \geq 1$.

10. GENERALIZATIONS

The flexibility of the framework of selective substitution grammars is once more demonstrated in the work of Siromoney and Subramanian [29] and of Siromoney and Dare [28]. In [29] selective substitution array grammars are introduced which provide a unifying framework for many of the two dimensional array grammars in the literature. In [28] a method is presented to generate infinite words using selective substitution grammars. This method is compared with some well-known ways of defining languages of infinite words. Relations between several infinitary language families obtained from selective substitution grammars are established and closure properties and decidability questions are studied.

11. GRAMMARS AND AUTOMATA

In formal language theory one can distinguish next to the grammatical approach an automata based approach to the study of formal languages. As with grammars numerous instances of automata have been defined in the literature. By singling out basic features of automata one may construct a framework for a general theory of automata. However, such a close look at automata may also lead to the insight that grammars and automata are very closely related. Such considerations have motivated the introduction of a unifying framework for grammars and automata. In Rozenberg [24] coordinated table selective substitution systems (cts systems, for short) were introduced as a unifying framework for both grammars and automata. This framework is an extension of the framework of s-grammars and is based on the rewriting of vectors of words rather than single words. Here we discuss a simplified version of cts systems. For the full framework and an extensive number of examples the reader is referred to [24].

A cts system is a construct $H = (G_1,\ldots G_n;R)$, $n \geq 1$, where, for $1 \leq i \leq n$, $G_i = (V_i,h_i,S_i,T_i,K_i)$ is an s-grammar, and R is a set of rewrites each of which is of the form $U = (U_1,\ldots,U_n)$ with $U_i \subseteq \{(a,w):w \in h_i(a) \text{ and } a \in V_i\}$. Hence, for each $1 \leq i \leq n$, U_i is a subset of the set of productions defined by h_i.
Given $x = (x_1,\ldots,x_n)$ and $y = (y_1,\ldots y_n)$ where $x_i,y_i \in V_i^*$, for $1 \leq i \leq n$, we say that x directly derives (or computes) y in H (using the rewrite U), denoted by $x \Rightarrow_H y$, if for every $1 \leq i \leq n$, x_i directly derives y_i in G_i using productions from U_i only. The reflexive and transitive closure of $\Rightarrow_H$ is denoted by $\overset{*}{\Rightarrow}_H$. The language L(H) of H is defined by
$L(H) = \{w \in T_1^* : (S_1,\ldots,S_n) \overset{*}{\Rightarrow}_H (w,\Lambda,\ldots,\Lambda)\}$.
In [24] various ways of defining languages of cts systems are discussed. One can interpretate one dimensional cts systems as (s-) grammars and more dimensional systems as automata with the first component as input and the other components as auxiliary (e.g., storage) devices. This motivates the above definition: a computation has ended only if the storage is empty.
Until now especially the following types of s-grammars have been used in the framework of cts systems.

Let $G = (V,h,S,T,K)$ be an s-grammar
G is RL, if *base*(G) $\in$ RLIN and $K = T^* \overline{(V-T)}$;
G is RB, if *base*(G) $\in$ EOS and $K = V^*\overline{V}$;
G is OL, if *base*(G) $\in$ EOS and $K = \overline{V}^*$;
G is OS, if *base*(G) $\in$ EOS and $K = V^*\overline{V}V^*$;
G is OS^2, if *base*(G) $\in$ EOS and $K = V^*\overline{VV}V^*$.
The class of cts systems $H = (G_1,\ldots,G_n;R)$ with G_i of type X_i, where $X_i \in \{RL,RB,OL,OS,OS^2\}$, for $1 \leq i \leq n$, is denoted by $(X_1,\ldots,X_n)$. The families of languages generated by cts systems from $(X_1,\ldots,X_n)$ are denoted by $\mathcal{L}_n(X_1,\ldots,X_n)$.

As in the framework of s-grammars one can investigate various families of selectors and their influence on the families of languages generated by cts systems using these selectors. In cts systems selectors can be used in a "direct mode" (on the first coordinate) and in an "indirect mode" (on another coordinate). In [24] it has been shown that the relative power of a family of selectors depends on the mode in which the selectors are used.

Theorem 11.1. $L_1(\mathrm{RB}) = L(\mathrm{Reg})$, $L_1(\mathrm{OS}) = L(\mathrm{EOS}) = L(\mathrm{CF})$, and $L_1(\mathrm{OL}) = L(\mathrm{EOL})$. □

This implies that $L_1(\mathrm{RB}) \subset L_1(\mathrm{OS}) \subset L_1(\mathrm{OL})$. If we use the same families of selectors at the second coordinate, the situation changes as can be seen from the next theorem. In all three cases we assume that the first component is RL which corresponds to the standard use of an input tape. $L(\mathrm{PN})$ in the statement of the theorem denotes the family of languages defined by labelled marked Petri nets with final zero marking (see Aalbersberg and Rozenberg [1]).

Theorem 11.2. $L_2(\mathrm{RL,RB}) = L(\mathrm{CF})$, $L_2(\mathrm{RL,OS}) = L(\mathrm{PN})$, and $L_2(\mathrm{RL,OL}) = L(\mathrm{Reg})$. □

This implies that $L_2(\mathrm{RL,OL}) \subset L_2(\mathrm{RL,RB})$, $L_2(\mathrm{RL,OL}) \subset L_2(\mathrm{RL,OS})$ and $L_2(\mathrm{RL,RB})$ and $L_2(\mathrm{RL,OS})$ are incomparable. The equality $L_2(\mathrm{RL,OS}) = L(\mathrm{PN})$ has been proved in Aalbersberg and Rozenberg [1]. In that paper the relationship between (classes of) Petri nets and (classes of) cts systems is investigated. In addition cts systems from $(\mathrm{RL,OS}^2)$ are investigated.

Theorem 11.3. $L_2(\mathrm{RL,OS}^2) = L(\mathrm{RE})$. □

It is interesting to compare this result with the remarks in Section 9 on $L_1(\mathrm{OS}^2) = L(p\{0^*110^*\})$.

The main part of the research in the framework of cts systems until now is devoted to (RL,RB) systems. (see Ehrenfeucht et al. [4] through [9]). (RL,RB) systems, usually called <u>coordinated pair systems</u> or cp <u>systems</u>, model the classical push-down automata (pda's for short). The notion of a cp system is simpler than that of a pda and the framework of cp systems gives rise to new results on the behaviour of pda's. Also new proofs for already known results can be provided without reference to other constructs like context-free grammars.

In [4] a normal form for cp systems is established yielding the so-called real-time cp systems. In the proof of this result rather than the grammatical Greibach normal form the structure of computations in cp systems is considered.
Much emphasis is given to the study of computations in cp systems. An important tool is the Exchange Theorem (see [7]) that describes how to swap subcomputations between computations in a cp system. In [8] and [9] this tool is used to investigate the possibilities of obtaining pumping properties of context-free languages via the analysis of computations in cp systems.
This leads in particular to an analysis of the structure of Dyck words. The correspondence between the structure of Dyck words and computations in cp systems can then be used to derive pumping lemma's. In [6] a survey of results is given.
In [5] the use of the "memory" (the RB component) of a cp system is investigated yielding as an overall conclusion that the evaluation of the memory behaviour depends strongly on the observation method chosen.

ACKNOWLEDGEMENT

The author is indebted to H.J. Hoogeboom for his careful reading of a first version of this paper.

REFERENCES

[1] Aalbersberg, IJ.J. and G. Rozenberg, CTS systems and Petri nets, *Theoretical Computer Science* 40 (1985), 149-162.

[2] Dahlhaus, E. and H. Gaifman, Concerning two-adjacent context-free languages, *Theoretical Computer Science* 41 (1985), 169-184.

[3] Dassow, J. and Gh. Păun, *Regulated rewriting in formal language theory*, in preparation.

[4] Ehrenfeucht, A., Hoogeboom, H.J., and G. Rozenberg, Real-time coordinated pair systems, Dept. of Comp. Sci., Univ. of Colorado at Boulder, Tech. Rep. CU-CS-259-83, 1983.

[5] Ehrenfeucht, A., Hoogeboom, H.J., and G. Rozenberg, On the active and full records of the use of memory in right-boundary grammars and push-down automata, *Theoretical Computer Science* 48 (1987) 201-228.

[6] Ehrenfeucht, A., Hoogeboom, H.J., and G. Rozenberg, On coordinated rewriting, *Lect. Notes in Comp. Sci.* 199 (1985), 100-111.

[7] Ehrenfeucht, A., Hoogeboom, H.J., and G. Rozenberg, Computations in coordinated pair systems, *Fundamentae Informaticae* IX (1986), 455-480.

[8] Ehrenfeucht, A., Hoogeboom, H.J., and G. Rozenberg, Coordinated pair systems. Part I: Dyck words and classical pumping, *R.A.I.R.O. Informatique Theorique* 20 (1986), 405-424.
[9] Ehrenfeucht, A., Hoogeboom, H.J., and G. Rozenberg, Coordinated pair systems. Part II: Sparse structure of Dyck words and Ogden's lemma, *R.A.I.R.O. Informatique Theorique* 20 (1986), 425-439.
[10] Ehrenfeucht, A., Kleijn, H.C.M., and G. Rozenberg, Adding global forbidding context to context-free grammars, *Theoretical Computer Science* 37 (1985), 337-360.
[11] Ehrenfeucht, A., Maurer, H., and G. Rozenberg, Continuous grammars, *Information and Control* 46 (1980), 71-91.
[12] Gonczarowski, J., Kleijn, H.C.M., and G. Rozenberg, Closure properties of selective substitution grammars. Part I, *International Journal of Computer Mathematics* 14 (1983), 19-42.
[13] Gonczarowski, J., Kleijn, H.C.M., and G. Rozenberg, Closure properties of selective substitution grammars. Part II, *International Journal of Computer Mathematics* 14 (1983), 109-134.
[14] Gonczarowski, J., Kleijn, H.C.M., and G. Rozenberg, Grammatical constructions in selective substitution grammars, *Acta Cybernetica* 6 (1983), 239-269.
[15] Gonczarowski, J. and E. Shamir, Pattern selector grammars and several parsing algorithms in the context-free style, *Journal of Computer and Systems Sciences* 30 (1985), 249-273.
[16] Gonczarowski, J. and M.K. Warmuth, Applications of scheduling theory to formal language theory, *Theoretical Computer Science* 37 (1985), 217-243.
[17] Kleijn, H.C.M., *Selective substitution grammars based on context-free productions*, Ph.D. Thesis, University of Leiden, 1983.
[18] Kleijn, H.C.M., and G. Rozenberg, Problems P 111-113, *EATCS Bulletin* 26 (1985), 240-241.
[19] Kleijn, H.C.M. and G. Rozenberg, Context-free like restrictions on selective rewriting, *Theoretical Computer Science* 16 (1981), 237-269.
[20] Kleijn, H.C.M. and G. Rozenberg, Sequential, continuous and parallel grammars, *Information and Control* 48 (1981), 221-260. Corrigendum, ibidem 52 (1982), 364.
[21] Kleijn, H.C.M. and G. Rozenberg, Multi grammars, *International Journal of Computer Mathematics* 12 (1983), 177-201.
[22] Kleijn, H.C.M. and G. Rozenberg, On the generative power of regular pattern grammars, *Acta Informatica* 20 (1983), 391-411.
[23] Rozenberg, G., Selective substitution grammars (Towards a framework for rewriting systems). Part I: Definitions and examples, *Elektronische Informationsverarbeitung und Kybernetik* 13 (1977), 455-463.
[24] Rozenberg, G., On coordinated selective substitutions: towards a unified theory of grammars and machines, *Theoretical Computer Science* 37 (1985), 31-50.
[25] Rozenberg, G. and A. Salomaa, *The mathematical theory of L systems*, Academic Press, New York, 1980.
[26] Rozenberg, G. and D. Wood, Context-free grammars with selective rewriting, *Acta Informatica* 13 (1980), 257-268.
[27] Salomaa, A., *Formal languages*, Academic Press, New York, 1973.
[28] Siromoney, R. and V.R. Dare, On infinite words obtained by selective substitution grammars, *Theoretical Computer Science* 39 (1985), 281-295.
[29] Siromoney, R. and K.G. Subramanian, Selective substitution array grammars, *Information Sciences* 25 (1981), 73-83.
[30] Subramanian, K.G., On the language class of continuous grammars, unpublished manuscript (1983).

SOME RECENT RESTRICTIONS
IN THE DERIVATION OF CONTEXT-FREE GRAMMARS

Gheorghe PĂUN
University of Bucharest
Faculty of Mathematics
Str. Academiei 14, 70109 Bucureşti
ROMANIA

We discuss here three classes of regulation mechanisms for context-free grammars, all three introduced in the eighties. The first one, the valence grammars in Păun /13/, associates numbers to production rules and accept as correct only derivations with a certain total valence. The second mechanism is a variant of random context restriction (strings instead of symbols in context sets) and it has been proposed by Kelemen /9/. The third restriction is a new one and it is based on the so-called walk language associated to a grammar.

1. Introduction

The regulated rewriting is a very rich in notions, results, problems and applications area of formal language theory. Proofs of this assertion can be found in the forthcoming monograph by Dassow, Păun /4/, where almost all the known regulation devices are presented.

The domain is not new: the first known restriction in derivation, the matrix one, already counts more than two decades (Abraham /1/). However, new restrictions still appear. We discuss here three of the recently introduced ones (definitions, examples, no-proof results, open problems). They are the valence grammars in Păun /13/, the semi-conditional grammars of Kelemen /9/ (see also Păun /14/) and the new, unpublished yet, walk restricted grammars.

The idea of this last regulation mechanism is the following:

take a context-free grammar and interpret the derivation process in an automata-type manner, that is consider a "rewriting head" which scans the current string and replaces certain nonterminals by right hand members of corresponding rules, then moves again and so on. The "walk" of this rewriting head can be described by a language, appropriately codifying the three basic actions it does: move to the right, move to the left, rewrite. Imposing restrictions to this language (to be given, as in a regular control grammar, for instance), we can obtain more variants of such a "walk restricted grammar". Generally, they have a great generative capacity (characterizations of context sensitive languages are obtained); some of them are strongly similar to the selective substitution grammars of Rozenberg (see Kleijn /10/ for detailed references).

In what follows, the reader is assumed familiar with formal language theory basic notions and results, including rudiments of regulated rewriting (see, for instance, Salomaa /17/). Some notations: V^* is the free monoid generated by V, λ is the unity of V^*, lg(x) is the length of x, RE, CS, CF, REG are the four families of languages in Chomsky hierarchy, LIN is the family of linear languages and MLIN is the family of metalinear ones. The components of a Chomsky grammar will be denoted $G = (V_N, V_T, S, P)$, with the nonterminals in V_N specified by capitals and the terminals in V_T by small letters.

2. Valence grammars

Definition 2.1. An additive valence grammar is a construct $G = (V_N, V_T, S, P, v)$, where $G' = (V_N, V_T, S, P)$ is a usual Chomsky grammar and $v : P \longrightarrow Z$ (Z is the set of integers). For a derivation

$$D : S \xrightarrow{r_1} w_1 \xrightarrow{r_2} \dots \xrightarrow{r_n} w_n$$

in G', we define

$$v(D) = \sum_{i=1}^{n} v(r_i)$$

The language generated by G is

$$L(G) = \{x \in V_T^* \,;\, D : S \overset{*}{\Longrightarrow} x \text{ in } G',\ v(D) = 0\}$$

Replacing Z by Q_+ (the set of positive rational numbers), the addition by multiplication and the condition $v(D) = 0$ by $v(D) = 1$, we obtain the <u>multiplicative valence grammars</u>.

<u>Example 2.1</u>. Consider the grammars G_i, $i = 1, 2$, identified by the next rules:

$r_1 : S \longrightarrow aS,\ v_1(r_1) = 1$ and	$r_1 : S \longrightarrow aS,\ v_2(r_1) = 2$
$r_2 : S \longrightarrow aA,\ v_1(r_2) = 0$	$r_2 : S \longrightarrow aA,\ v_2(r_2) = 1$
$r_3 : A \longrightarrow bA,\ v_1(r_3) = -1$	$r_3 : A \longrightarrow bA,\ v_2(r_3) = 3$
$r_4 : A \longrightarrow b,\ v_1(r_4) = 0$	$r_4 : A \longrightarrow bB,\ v_2(r_4) = 1$
	$r_5 : B \longrightarrow cB,\ v_2(r_5) = 1/6$
	$r_6 : B \longrightarrow c,\ v_2(r_6) = 1.$

We obtain

$$L(G_1) = \{a^n b^n \,;\, n \geq 1\} \quad \text{(additive valences)}$$
$$L(G_2) = \{a^n b^n c^n \,;\, n \geq 1\} \quad \text{(multiplicative valences)}$$

Denote by AV(X) (MV(X)) the families of languages generated by additive (multiplicative, respectively) valence grammars of type X, X a class in Chomsky hierarchy. The above examples show that AV(REG) contains non-regular languages and MV(REG) contains non-context-free languages. In what follows, REG stands for right-linear grammars and the grammars can possibly contain λ-rules.

The following results were proved in Păun /13/ (some new proofs are given in Dassow, Păun /4/) and in Gheorghe /6/:

THEOREM 2.1.

(i) The families AV(REG), MV(REG) can be characterized in terms of one-way nondeterministic finite automata with addition/multiplication and without equality in Ibarra et al. /8/.

(ii) The families MV(X) equal the families of unordered generalized vector grammars of type X in Cremers, Mayer /2/, /3/.

(iii) $X \subset AV(X) \subset MV(X)$, $X \in \{CF, LIN, REG\}$, strict inclusions.

(iv) $AV(REG) \subset AV(LIN) \subset AV(CF)$,

$MV(REG) \subset MV(LIN) \subset MV(CF)$,

$AV(REG) \subset CF$, strict inclusions.

(v) The families in the next pairs are incomparable:

AV(REG) and LIN, MV(REG) and CF,

MV(REG) and AV(CF), MV(REG) and LIN,

MV(REG) and MLIN, AV(LIN) and CF,

AV(LIN) and MLIN, MV(LIN) and CF.

Considering the above characterizations (and the results in Cremers, Mayer /2/, /3/ and in Ibarra et al. /8/) as well as by ad-hoc proofs, many closure properties were obtained for valence grammars. We do not discuss them here, but we present some results of Marcus, Păun /11/, concerning an extension of valence restriction to gsm mappings.

Definition 2.2. An additive valence gsm is a system $g = (K, I, O, s_0, F, P, v)$, where $g' = (K, I, O, s_0, F, P)$ is a usual gsm (with the moves in P specified as rewriting rules, $sa \longrightarrow xs'$, $s, s' \in K$, $a \in I$, $x \in O^*$) and $v : P \longrightarrow Z$. The valence $v(D)$ of some rewriting

$$D : ys_1a_1a_2\ldots a_nz \xRightarrow{r_1} yx_1s_2a_2\ldots a_nz \xRightarrow{r_2} \ldots$$

$$\ldots \xRightarrow{r_{n-1}} yx_1\ldots x_{n-1}s_na_nz \xRightarrow{r_n} yx_1\ldots x_ns_{n+1}z,$$

$z \in I^*$, $y \in O^*$, $r_i : s_ia_i \longrightarrow x_is_{i+1} \in P$, $1 \leq i \leq n$, is defined by

$$v(D) = \sum_{i=1}^{n} v(r_i)$$

and, for $w \in I^*$,

$$g(w) = \{z \in O^* \ ; \text{ there is } D : s_0w \xRightarrow{*} zs_f,\ s_f \in F,\ v(D) = 0\}$$

A similar definition holds for multiplicative valence gsm's: replace Z by Q_+, addition by multiplication and $v(D) = 0$ by $v(D) = 1$.

We denote by AGSM the class of additive valence gsm's, and by MGSM the class of multiplicative valence gsm's. By AGSM(X), MGSM(X) we denote the families of languages obtained by translating a language in the family X by mappings in AGSM, MGSM, respectively. Write

$AGSM^n(X)$, $MGSM^n(X)$ for n times iterated such translations.

The following results were proved in Marcus, Păun /11/:

THEOREM 2.2.

(i) $AV(X) = AGSM(X)$,

$MV(X) = MGSM(X)$, $X \in \{CF, LIN, REG\}$.

(In this way a new characterization of vector languages is obtained, as the image of context-free languages by multiplicative valence gsm mappings.)

(ii) The class AGSM is not closed under composition and the families $AV(X)$, $X \in \{CF, REG\}$, are not closed under additive valence gsm mappings.

(iii) The class MGSM is closed under composition (therefore $MV(X)$, $X \in \{CF, REG\}$, are closed under multiplicative valence gsm mappings).

(iv) $MGSM^n(X) = MGSM(X)$, $n \geq 1$, $X \in \{CF, REG\}$,

$AGSM^n(REG)$, $n \geq 2$, are incomparable with CF,

$AGSM^n(X) \subseteq MGSM(X)$, $n \geq 1$, $X \in \{CF, REG\}$.

Open problems:

Q1. Which are the relations between MLIN and AV(REG), MV(LIN) ?

Q2. The families $AGSM^n(X)$, $n \geq 1$, $X \in \{CF, REG\}$, define two hierarchies which lie in between AV(X) and MV(X). Are these hierarchies infinite ? We expect an affirmative answer.

Q3. Here we considered valence grammars (and gsm's) involving the particular groups $(Z, +, 0)$ and $(Q_+, \cdot, 1)$. What about considering arbitrary groups ? For instance, can we obtain an infinite hierarchy of language families taking the groups $(Z^n, +, (0, 0, \dots, 0))$, $n \geq 1$? Denote by $AV_n(X)$, $n \geq 1$, $X \in \{CF, REG\}$, the family of languages generated by additive valence grammars of the form $G = (V_N, V_T, S, P, v)$ $v : P \longrightarrow Z^n$. We obtain (Gheorghe, Păun /7/):

(i) $AV(X) = AV_1(X)$,

(ii) $AV_n(X) \subseteq AV_{n+1}(X)$, $n \geq 1$,

(iii) $\bigcup_{n \geq 1} AV_n(X) = MV(X)$, $X \in \{CF, REG\}$,

therefore the hierarchies $AV_n(X)$ lie in between $AV(X)$ and $MV(X)$, $X \in \{CF, REG\}$, respectively. We feel that these hierarchies are infinite too.

3. Semi-conditional grammars

Kelemen /9/ has proposed the following type of regulated mechanism, with AI motivation: add to each rule $A \longrightarrow x$ in a given grammar $G = (V_N, V_T, S, P)$ a string w over $V_G = V_N \cup V_T$ and apply this rule only for rewriting strings which have w as substring. Such a restriction is similar to the conditional one (Friš /5/, Păun /12/), where a language is added to each rule and the rule is applied to strings in the associated language, as well as to random context grammars (Van der Walt /18/), in which each rule has a set Q of permitting symbols and a set R of forbidding symbols, the rule being applied only to strings which contain all symbols in Q and no symbol in R. A generalization of Kelemen grammars were considered in Păun /14/, under the name of semi-conditional grammars.

Definition 3.1. Let i, j be two natural numbers. A semi-conditional grammar of degree (i, j) is a system $G = (V_N, V_T, S, P)$, where V_N, V_T, S are as in a usual grammar and P is a finite set of production rules of the form $(A \longrightarrow x, z_1, z_2)$, where $A \longrightarrow x$ is a context-free rule, z_1 is missing or $z_1 \in V_G^*$, $lg(z_1) \leq i$, and z_2 is missing or $z_2 \in V_G^*$, $lg(z_2) \leq j$. Such a rule can be applied to a string w if and only if z_1 (if z_1 is not missing) is a substring of w and z_2 (if z_2 is not missing) is not a substring of w. (When both z_1, z_2 are missing, then the rule can be applied without restrictions.)

We denote by $SK(i, j)$, $i \geq 0$, $j \geq 0$, the family of languages generated by λ-free context-free semi-conditional grammars of degree (i, j); when λ-rules are allowed, a superscript λ is added.

The following results were proved in Păun /14/:

THEOREM 3.1.

(i) Both families SK(1, 0), SK(0, 1) contain non-semilinear languages, hence they include strictly the family CF.

(ii) $SK(1, 1) \subset CS$, strict inclusion.

(iii) $SK(2, 1) = CS = SK(1, 2)$,

$SK^{\lambda}(2, 1) = RE = SK^{\lambda}(1, 2)$.

(iv) $SK_{left}(1, 0) = CS = SK_{left}(0, 2)$,

$SK^{\lambda}_{left}(1, 0) = RE = SK^{\lambda}_{left}(0, 2)$

(the subscript left indicates the restriction to leftmost derivations in the usual sense).

To a semi-conditional grammar one can impose a further regulating device, for instance, the order restriction of Friš /5/ (introduce a partial order of rules and use the maximal applicable rules for rewriting the current string), the programmed restriction (Rozenkrantz /15/), the regular control (Salomaa /16/) or the matrix restriction (Abraham /1/). We shall add the letters O, P, C, M in the front of SK(i, j) in order to denote the corresponding families of languages, respectively. As it is expected, new characterizations of CS and RE families are obtained in this way. Please note that we do not use appearance checking features in programmed ($\varphi(r) = \emptyset$ for all rules), regular control and matrix grammars ($F = \emptyset$).

THEOREM 3.2.

$XSK(2, 0) = CS = XSK(0, 2)$, $X \in \{O, P, M, C\}$,

$XSK^{\lambda}(2, 0) = RE = XSK^{\lambda}(0, 2)$, $X \in \{O, P, M, C\}$.

A similar result can be obtained also when considering the semi-conditional restriction imposed to matrix grammars (matrices with an associated pair (z_1, z_2) as above; the whole matrix is applied only to strings containing z_1 and not containing z_2, when z_1, z_2 are not missing).

Also for this regulation mechanism some problems have remained open:

Q4. Are SK(i, 0), SK(0, i), $i \geq 2$, strictly included into CS ? (Remember points (ii) and (iii) of Theorem 3.1.) Is $SK_{left}(0, 1)$ strictly included into CS ?

Q5. Are the inclusions $SK(1, 0) \subseteq SK(1, 1)$, $SK(0, 1) \subseteq SK(1, 1)$ proper ? Which relations there are between SK(0, i) and SK(i, 0), $i \geq 1$?

4. Walk restricted grammars

Consider a context-free grammar $G = (V_N, V_T, S, P)$. When in some string $w = x_1Ax_2Bx_3$ we first rewrite the A occurrence and then the B occurrence, we can say that the "writing head" of the grammar has moved from A to B. We can thus think in terms of automata even when dealing with grammars. We shall formalize this in the following way:

Definition 4.1. Let $G = (V_N, V_T, S, P)$ be a context-free grammar and consider a derivation D according to G,

$$D : S = w_0 \Longrightarrow w_1 \Longrightarrow \dots \Longrightarrow w_n \in V_T^*$$

The "grammar scanner" is initially positioned on S and for w_j, $j \geq 1$, it is positioned according to the next rules:

1. If $w_i \Longrightarrow w_{i+1}$, $w_i = x_1Ax_2$, $w_{i+1} = x_1yzx_2$, $x_1, y, x_2 \in V_G^*$, $z \in V_G$, and the scanner is positioned on A in w_i, then the scanner is positioned on z in w_{i+1}.
2. If $w_i \Longrightarrow w_{i+1}$ as above, the used rule was $A \longrightarrow \lambda$ and the scanner is positioned on A in w_i, then in w_{i+1} the scanner is positioned on z in $x_2 = zx_2'$ when $x_2 \neq \lambda$, or on z in $x_1 = x_1'z$ when $x_2 = \lambda$, $x_1 \neq \lambda$; the scanner is "lost" when $w_{i+1} = \lambda$.

The "walk" of the grammar scanner can be codified as follows. If, according to the above definition, the scanner is positioned on z in w_i, $w_i = y_1zy_2Ax_2$, and this occurrence of A is rewritten in

$w_i \Longrightarrow w_{i+1}$, then we say that the scanner has been moved k steps to the right, $k = lg(y_2A)$. When $w_i = x_1Ay_1zy_2$ we say that the scanner has been moved k steps to the left, $k = lg(Ay_1)$.

Let us denote by 0 the action of rewriting (using a rule), by 1 the scanner moving for a step to the right and by 2 the scanner moving for a step to the left. We write

$$walk(w_i, D) = 1^k, \quad walk(w_i, D) = 2^k$$

in the above cases, respectively. Thus, the scanner walk (including the rewritings) in the derivation D will be described by the string

$$walk(D) = 0\ walk(w_1, D)\ 0\ walk(w_2, D) \ldots 0\ walk(w_{n-1}, D)\ 0$$

In this way, a language

$$walk(G) = \{walk(D)\ ;\ D \text{ is a derivation in } G\}$$

can be associated to the grammar G.

Example 4.1. Clearly, if G is a linear grammar, then walk(G) is a regular sublanguage of $\{0, 2\}^*$.

Take now the metalinear grammar G with the rules

$$S \longrightarrow AB,\ A \longrightarrow Aa,\ B \longrightarrow bB,\ A \longrightarrow a,\ B \longrightarrow b$$

We have

$$L(G) = \{a^nb^m\ ;\ n, m \geq 1\}$$

$$walk(G) \cap 0(2^+01^+0)^* = \{020102^301^30 \ldots 2^{2k+1}01^{2k+1}0\ ;\ k \geq 1\}$$

therefore the language walk(G) is not context-free.

It is easy to see that the language walk(G) is context sensitive for each context-free grammar G. As the language walk(G) is similar in some sense with the Szilard language associated to G, it might be interesting to examine it as a goal per se. We shall not insist on this direction here, but we shall define a regulating mechanism on this basis (in the same way as the regular control grammars are defined starting from Szilard languages).

Definition 4.2. A regular walk grammar is a system $G = (V_N, V_T, S, P, C)$, where $G' = (V_N, V_T, S, P)$ is a usual context-free grammar and C is a regular language over $\{0, 1, 2\}$. The language L(G) is

$$L(G) = \{x \in V_T^* \ ; \text{ there is a derivation } D : S \overset{*}{\Longrightarrow} x \text{ in } G' \text{ such that walk}(D) \in C\}$$

We denote by RW the family of languages generated by regular walk λ-free context-free grammars; when λ-rules are allowed, we write RW^{λ}.

The inclusions

$$RW \subseteq CS, \quad RW^{\lambda} \subseteq RE$$

can be proved by a standard construction. The following examples will show that the inclusion $CF \subset RW$ is proper (moreover, RW contains non-semilinear languages).

<u>Example 4.2</u>. Consider the grammar G with the rules

$$S \longrightarrow AB, \ A \longrightarrow aAb, \ B \longrightarrow cB, \ A \longrightarrow ab, \ B \longrightarrow c$$

and with the regular language

$$C = 02(01^+02^+)^*$$

It is easy to see that all correct terminal derivations must be of the form

$$S \Longrightarrow AB \Longrightarrow aAbB \Longrightarrow aAbcB \Longrightarrow a^2Ab^2cB \Longrightarrow a^2Ab^2c^2B \Longrightarrow \ldots$$
$$\ldots \Longrightarrow a^nAb^nc^nB \Longrightarrow a^{n+1}b^{n+1}c^nB \Longrightarrow a^{n+1}b^{n+1}c^{n+1}$$

hence

$$L(G) = \{a^nb^nc^n \ ; \ n \geq 1\}$$

<u>Example 4.3</u>. Consider the grammar G with the rules

$$S \longrightarrow BAAc, \ B \longrightarrow bB, \ B \longrightarrow b, \ A \longrightarrow AAc, \ A \longrightarrow a$$

and with the regular language

$$C = 02^3(00(1^+0)^+2^+)^*$$

Let us remark that the substrings 00 of strings in C imply the use of rules $B \longrightarrow bB$, $B \longrightarrow b$ (after using $A \longrightarrow AAc$ the scanner is positioned on c). Moreover, after using two times the rule $B \longrightarrow bB$ (thus introducing two occurrences of b), the scanner goes to the right and at least a rewriting is performed (the substring 1^+0); then we return to the left symbol B and the process is reiterated. In consequence, the strings in L(G) are of the form $b^{2n}w$ with $w \in \{a, c\}^*$, $n + 1 \leq lg_a(w) \leq$

$\leqslant 2^n$, $n \leqslant lg_c(w) \leqslant 2^n - 1$ ($lg_z(w)$ is the number of symbol z occurrences in the string w). This language is not semilinear.

Some variants of the walk restricted grammars could be of interest. For instance, instead of 0 in the walk control language we can consider a nonterminal; the rewriting specified by 0 must now consists of rewriting the corresponding nonterminal. Another possibility is to replace 0 by a production rule label and to use this rule at the corresponding step of a derivation.

Example 4.4. Consider a context sensitive grammar G in Kuroda normal form and let r : $AB \longrightarrow CD$ be a rewriting rule in G. Construct a context-free regular walk grammar G' introducing the associated rules

$$A \longrightarrow A_r,\ A_r \longrightarrow C,\ B \longrightarrow B_r,\ B_r \longrightarrow D$$

and considering the string AA_r1BB_r (instead of 00100) as a substring of the associated walk control language. Clearly, in this way the grammar G' can simulate the rule r, hence we obtain L(G) = L(G').

A similar result is true for the case when we replace the 0 occurrences by rule labels, therefore these variants of walk restricted grammars characterize the context sensitive languages (recursively enumerable languages, when λ-rules are used).

Of course, the study of walk restricted grammars needs much further efforts. Here are some open problems and research topics which seem to deserve our attention:

Q6. Is the inclusion $RW \subseteq CS$ a proper one ? Compare the family RW with other families obtained by regulated rewriting.

Q7. What about considering a context-free walk language ? What about adding appearance checking features ? (Mark some occurrences of 0 in the stringsof the walk language C and use them in the appearance checking manner, that is ignore them when no rewriting is possible in this place.)

References

1. S. Abraham, Some questions of phrase-structure grammars, Comput. Lingv., 4 (1965), 61 - 70.

2. A.B. Cremers, O. Mayer, On matrix languages, Inform. Control, 23 (1973), 86 - 96.

3. A.B. Cremers, O. Mayer, On vector languages, Proc. Symp. Summer School Math. Found. Comp. Sci., High Tatras, 1973.

4. J. Dassow, Gh. Păun, The regulated rewriting in formal language theory, Akademie Verlag, Berlin (in press).

5. I. Friš, Grammars with partial ordering of rules, Inform. Control, 12 (1968), 415 - 425.

6. M. Gheorghe, Linear valence grammars, Proc. 4th Intern. Meeting Young Comp. Sci., Smolenice, 1986.

7. M. Gheorghe, Gh. Păun, Two (infinite ?) hierarchies of vector languages, Bull. of the EATCS, 29 (1986), 27 - 32.

8. O.H. Ibarra, S.K. Sahni, C.E. Kim, Finite automata with multiplication, Th. Comp. Sci., 2 (1976), 271 - 294.

9. J. Kelemen, Conditional grammars. Motivations, definition and some properties, Proc. Conf. Aut. Lang. Math. Syst., Salgotarjan, 1984.

10. J. Kleijn, Selective substitution grammars based on context-free productions, Doctoral Dissertation, Univ. of Leiden, 1983.

11. M. Marcus, Gh. Păun, Valence gsm mappings, Bull. Math. Soc. Sci. Math. R.S. Roumanie (in press).

12. Gh. Păun, On the generative capacity of conditional grammars, Inform. Control, 43 (1979), 178 - 186.

13. Gh. Păun, A new generative device: valence grammars, Rev. Roum. Math. Pures Appl., 25 (1980), 911 - 924.

14. Gh. Păun, A variant of random context grammars: semi-conditional grammars, Th. Comp. Sci., 41 (1985), 1 - 17.

15. D. Rozenkrantz, Programmed grammars and classes of formal languages, Journal of the ACM, 16 (1969), 107 - 131.

16. A. Salomaa, On some families of formal languages obtained by regulated derivations, Ann. Acad. Sci. Fenn., Ser. A1, 1970, 479.

17. A. Salomaa, Formal languages, Academic Press, New York, London,1973.

18. A.P.J. Van der Walt, Random context languages, Symp. on Formal Languages at the MFI Oberwolfach, 1970, North-Holland, 1972, 66 - 68.

Chapter 3

BIOLOGICALLY MOTIVATED STRUCTURES

RECENT RESULTS ON THE THEORY OF HOMOGENEOUS STRUCTURES

Victor Aladyev
SKB MPSM ESSR, Tallinn 200035
Paldiski mnt 171-26

1. INTRODUCTION

The homogeneous structure(HS) is an information parallel processing system consisting of intercommunicating identical finite automata. Although "homogeneous structures" will be the usual term throughout this work, it should be borne in mind that "cellular automata" and so on are essentially synonymous. We can interpret HS as theoretical framework of artificial parallel information processing systems. From the logical point of view the HS is a infinite automaton with characteristic internal structure. The theory of HS can be considered to be the structural and dynamic theory of the infinite automata. HS can serve as the basis for modelling of many discrete processes and they present enough interesting independent objects of investigations as well. HS can serve as a formal model of parallel computations, the same as Turing machine is formal model of the modern concept of computability. During the recent years there has been considerable interest in the theory of HS about which many interesting results have been obtained. Much of this work has been motivated by the growing interest in computer science and biological modelling.

In our previous works [1-5,9,10] we investigated different aspects of the HS theory and their applications in computer science and biological modelling. Results in this directions contributed much that is new to the HS theory and its applications. However, many questions still remained open in the present topic. In this work we present our recent solutions of a number of open questions in the HS theory. This work is organized so as to discuss the more general problems and results obtained therein. It is rather unfortunate that we have no space here to discuss in detail the basic techniques for solving problems. Exhaustive information about these can be found in Aladyev[6-8]. The all general terms, notions and designations are given in item 2 or are well-known enough. All the others are introduced as the necessity arises.

2. GENERAL DEFINITIONS, CONCEPTS AND NOTIONS

The classical d-dimensional HS(d-HS) is an ordered set of four components

$$d\text{-HS}=\langle Z^d, A, \tau^{(n)}, X\rangle,$$

where $A=\{0,1,2,\dots,a-1\}$ is a set called the state alphabet of the individual finite automata in the structure. Z^d is the set of all d-tuples of integers which is used to name the cell, where Z is the set of integers and is called the array. Each cell z in Z^d can be thought of as the name or address of the particular automaton which occupies that position in the array. X, called the neighbourhood index of the d-HS, is an n-tuple of distinct d-tuples of integers and is used to define the neighbours of any cell, i.e., those cells from which the cell z will directly receive information. The neighbourhood index X describes the uniform interconnection pattern(template) among the automata in the d-HS($d\geq 1$). The first three above-mentioned components of any d-HS, namely, A, Z^d and X, form a homogeneous space. The state of the entire space is called a configuration(CF) of the space and is any mapping CF: $Z^d \rightarrow A$, null-CF($\overline{0}$) is a mapping $\overline{0}$: $Z^d \rightarrow 0$. C_A denotes the set of all CF with respect to Z^d and A, i.e., $C_A=\{CF \mid CF: Z^d \rightarrow A\}$. Let c(z) be the current state of the machine located at cell z. The support of a CF c is the set of all cells z such that $c(z)\neq 0$, i.e., the support is the nonquiescent part of CF c. CF with finite support are of considerable interest; the set of all such CF is denoted by $\overline{C}_A$. The set of all infinite CF of d-HS is denoted by $\overset{\infty}{C}_A$; obviously, that $\overline{C}_A \cup \overset{\infty}{C}_A = C_A$ and $\overline{C}_A \cap \overset{\infty}{C}_A = \emptyset$.

The operation of the d-HS is specified by a local function $\sigma^{(n)}$ which produces the next state of an individual automaton z in terms of the states of the automata which are directly connected to z. In This work we shall be concerned, in general, with a local function, which is defined to be a mapping from A^n to A such that $\sigma^{(n)}(0^n)$ always equals 0. The d-HS with such local function is called a stable. For the rest, a local function is any mapping $\sigma^{(n)}: A^n \rightarrow A$.

The simultaneous application of a local function $\sigma^{(n)}$ to the neighbourhood of every cell of the homogeneous space defines a global function $\tau^{(n)}$ of the current CF c into the next CF c $\tau^{(n)}$. The operation of a d-HS is particularly simple. If $c=c_0$ is an initial CF of the homogeneous space at time t=0, then the CF at time t=m is $c_0 \tau^{(n)m}$, the result of applying $\tau^{(n)}$ to the homogeneous space m times. Let $\langle c_0\rangle[\tau^{(n)}]$ denote the CF-sequence generated by function $\tau^{(n)}$ from the CF $c_0 \in C_A$. Now we define the nonconstructibility in d-HS($d \geqslant 1$). Questions of nonconstructibility are fundamental problems in the study of the theoretical properties of the d-HS.

<u>Definition 1.</u> CF c is nonconstructible(NCF) for function $\tau^{(n)}$ of d-HS($d \geqslant 1$) iff there does not exist CF $c_o \in C_A$ such that CF $c_o \tau^{(n)}$ contains CF c as subconfiguration.

<u>Definition 2.</u> CF $c \in \overline{C}_A$ is called NCF-1 for function $\tau^{(n)}$ of d-HS iff there exists CF $c' \in \overline{C}_A$ such that $c' \tau^{(n)} = c$ and there does not exist CF $c^x \in \overline{C}_A$ such that $c^x \tau^{(n)} = c$.

<u>Definition 3.</u> Two CF $c_1, c_2 \in \overline{C}_A$ form for function $\tau^{(n)}$ a pair of the mutually erasable CF(MEC) iff $c_1 \tau^{(n)} = c_2 \tau^{(n)}$.

Each d-HS($d \geqslant 1$) can be assumed as a parallel formal τ_n-grammar with an axiom $c_o \in \overline{C}_A$(initial CF in d-HS) and productions $\tau^{(n)}$(global function of d-HS). L(τ_n)-language is the set of all words that can be derived from axiom c_o by means of applications of global function $\tau^{(n)}$.

The general decomposition problem(GDP) of global functions in the d-HS($d \geqslant 1$) can be presented as follows: Can any global function $\tau^{(n)}$ of d-HS be presented in the form of composition of the finite number of more simple global functions $\tau^{(n_i)}(n_i < n;\ i=\overline{1,k})$?

Within the framework of the classical d-HS can be selected some special subclasses of structures with specific properties: d-HS with refractority, memory and so on, which allow to design a number of interesting phenomena and processes[12].

Now we shall discuss the most significant, in our opinion, recent results in the HS theory and their applications. This work we have done over the years 1984-86 and the first quarter of 1986[6-13].

3. GENERAL RESULTS

Above all, we turn one's eyes again upon the GDP of global functions in d-HS. The GDP was solved by Aladyev[2] with the help on nonconstructibility approach in d-HS. In our works[3,4] the GDP received further decisions on the basis of other interesting approaches, in the first place, with the help of Shannon's function and on the basis of results in the K-valued logics($K \geqslant 2$). On a level with well-known GDP it is interesting to investigate the so-called global decomposition problem(GLDP) of global functions of d-HS($d \geqslant 1$). The GLDP is the question whether or not any global function $\tau^{(n)}$ of d-HS will possess the following representation:

$$\tau^{(n)} = \tau_1^{(n1)}\ \tau_2^{(n_2)} \ldots\ldots\ \tau_k^{(n_k)} \qquad (1)$$

This means that we may use arbitrary global functions as functions $\tau_i^{(n_i)}$ $(i=\overline{1,k})$ in representation (1). Clearly, the positive solution of the GDP for function $\tau^{(n)}$ entail the positive solution of the GLDP for this global function. The inverse assertion is not true, broadly speaking. Therefore, the GDP and the GLDP are not equivalent, generally. In connection with the GLDP Aladyev[6] proved the following result.

<u>Theorem 1.</u> The GLDP for global functions $\tau^{(n)}$ has negative solution, in general.

<u>Theorem 2.</u> If for some global function $\tau^{(n)}$ the GDP and the GLDP are equivalent, then for this function these problems are decidable.

The utilization of possibility of representation of local function $\sigma^{(n)}$ in the form of polynomial in modulo a(a - prime) allow to receive the following interesting result.

<u>Theorem 3.</u> For any global function $\tau^{(n)}$ in alphabet $A_p=\{0,1,2,3,4,\ldots,a-1\}$(a - prime) the GDP and the GLDP are equivalent, and algorithmically decidable.

Theorem 3 gives answers on a number of problems from our book[10]. Furthermore, theorems 2 and 3 show that structure of alphabet A of the d-HS has of vital importance for the equivalence of the GDP and the GLDP. Using now theorem 3 and proof of theorem 1 the following theorem can be proved.

<u>Theorem 4.</u> The GDP and the GLDP for function $\tau^{(n)}$ in alphabet A_p have positive solutions iff the function $\tau^{(n)}$ can be presented in the form of composition $\tau^{(n)} = \tau^{(m)}\ \tau^{(q)}$ $(m,q<n;\ m+q-1=n)$ of two functions in the same alphabet.

From theorem 4 the following interesting result may be drawn.

<u>Theorem 5.</u> For any integer $n \geqslant 3$ there exist functions $\tau^{(n)}$ in alphabet A_p for which the GDP and the GLDP are equivalent and have negative solutions.

This theorem present just one more proof of negative solutions of the GDP and the GLDP. Using the proof of theorem 5, we can to estimate the quota of functions $\tau^{(n)}$ in alphabet A_p for which the GDP and the GLDP have positive solutions.

<u>Theorem 6.</u> The GDP and the GLDP for "almost all" functions $\tau^{(n)}$ in alphabet A_p have negative solutions.

Thus, we received slightly unexpected result, namely: quota of all functions $\tau^{(n)}$ $(n \geqslant 3)$ in alphabet A_p, which have positive solutions of the GDP and the GLDP, is equal to zero. From Aladyev's results[6] on the GDP and the GLDP, it can be easily verified that among all functions $\tau^{(n)}$ $(n\geqslant 2)$ in alphabet A_p the infinite hierarchy of complexity with respect to the GDP/GLDP can be established. We shall say that function $\tau^{(n)}$ in alphabet A_p belongs to p-level of complexity(denotion: $\tau^{(n)}\in L(p)$) iff for it there exists representation

$$\tau^{(n)} = \tau_1^{(n_1)} \ \ldots\ldots \ \tau_k^{(n_k)} \qquad (n_i \leqslant p < n; (\exists\, i)(n_i = p); i=\overline{1,k})$$

and there does not exist representation of the similar type with $n_i > p$ $(i=\overline{1,k})$. If the GDP(GLDP) for function $\tau^{(n)}$ has negative solution, then $\tau^{(n)}\in L(n)$. Using the above-mentioned results on the GDP and the GLDP, and the proof of theorem 6 we can receive the following correlations:

$$(\forall p\geqslant 2)(\neq\neq L(p)\neq 0) \qquad \lim_{p\to\infty} \neq\neq L(p)/a^{a^p} \geqslant 1 \ (a - \text{prime})$$

From theorem 3 and the definition of complexity with respect to the GDP/GLDP of global functions $\tau^{(n)}$ the following result can be drawn.

<u>Theorem 7.</u> The problem of determination of p-level of complexity with respect to the GDP/GLDP for arbitrary global function $\tau^{(n)}$ in alphabet A_p is algorithmically decidable.

In view of definition of complexity with respect to the GDP/GLDP of functions $\tau^{(n)}$, Aladyev[6-8] received a number of characteristics of global functions depending on their complexity. From above-mentioned results(theorems 3-7) it is clear that we essentially used the alphabet A_p, since the local function $\sigma^{(n)}$ in this alphabet can be presented in the form of polynomial in modulo a of maximal degree n(a-1) over field A_p, and vice versa. In the case of composite integer a far from each function $\sigma^{(n)}$ in alphabet A can be presented in the polynomial form, generally speaking.

<u>Theorem 8.</u> For each alphabet $A=\{0,1,2,\ldots,a-1\}$(a - composite integer) the quota h of local functions in the alphabet A, which are presented in the form of polynomial in modulo a, satisfy the correlation

$$1/a^{a^n-4^n} \leqslant h \leqslant 1/a^{a^n-(a-2)^n}$$

Theorem 8 shows that for composite integers a "almost all" local functions $\sigma^{(n)}$ in alphabet A cannot be presented in the form of polynomial in modulo a for enough large integers n or/and a. Aladyev[10] formulated the following problem: Is it possible to define the algebraical system, which permit the polynomial representation of local functions for case of composite integer a, like of the case of prime a Various algebraical systems have been proposed to answer this question

We present now an algebraical system in which "almost all" local functions in alphabet A(a - composite integer) has representation in the form of polynomial in modulo a. We define the system in the following way. Let on the set $A=\{0,1,\dots,a-1\}$ (a - composite integer) the usual operation (+) of addition in modulo a is defined. At the same time, on the set A the binary operation of $\otimes$-multiplication is introduced in conformity with the following table

$$\begin{array}{c|ccccccccc} \otimes & 0 & 1 & 2 & 3 & 4 & 5 & \dots & (a-1) \\ 0 & 0 & 0 & 0 & 0 & 0 & 0 & \dots & 0 \\ 1 & 0 & 1 & 2 & 3 & 4 & 5 & \dots & (a-1) \\ 2 & 0 & 2 & 3 & 4 & 5 & 6 & \dots & 1 \\ 3 & 0 & 3 & 4 & 5 & 6 & 7 & \dots & 12 \\ 4 & 0 & 4 & 5 & 6 & 7 & 8 & \dots & 123 \\ 5 & 0 & 5 & 6 & 7 & 8 & 9 & \dots & 1234 \\ \dots & \dots & \dots & \dots & \dots & \dots & \dots & \dots & \dots \\ a-1 & 0 & (a-1) & \dots & 4 & & & \dots & (a-3)(a-2) \end{array} \qquad (2)$$

It can be easily seen that operation $\otimes$-multiplication on the set $A\setminus\{0\}$ form the finite cyclic group $A^{\otimes}$ of degree (a-1). In view of our above-mentioned suppositions the following general result can be established.

<u>Theorem 9.</u> There exist an algebraical system $\langle A; +; \otimes\rangle$ in which "almost each" local function $\sigma^{(n)}$ in the alphabet A can be unequivocally presented in the form of polynomical $P_{\otimes}(n)$ (mod a), where:

1. (+) is operation of addition in modulo a, which form on the set A the finite additive cyclic group of degree a;
2. ($\otimes$) is operation of $\otimes$-multiplication, which is determined by table (2) and which form on the set $A\setminus\{0\}$ the finite cyclic group of degree (a-1);
3. polynomial $P_{\otimes}(n) = \sum_{1}^{a^n-1} c_i \otimes X_1^{k_{i_1}} \otimes X_2^{k_{i_2}} \otimes \dots \otimes X_n^{k_{i_n}} \pmod a$ contains no binomials of the form $P_k X_j^k + B_k X_j^{a-k-1}$

$$(0 \leqslant k_{i_j} \leqslant a-1;\ \sum_{j}^{n} k_{i_j} \geqslant 1;\ X_j, c_i \in A;\ j=\overline{1,n};\ i=\overline{1,a^n-1}; \qquad (3)$$
$$P_k + B_k = a;\ P_k, B_k \geqslant 1;\ k=\overline{1,[(a-2)/2]}).$$

Theorem 9 plays a very important role in investigations of dynamic properties of d-HS($d \geqslant 1$) in the case of alphabet $A=\{0,1,\dots,a-1\}$ for composite integer a. Furthermore, the theorem gives comfortable analytical representation of functions of a-valued logics in the case of composite integer a. To our knowledge this result is the best of its kind. Using now the proofs of theorems 2 and 3, and the result of theorem 9, it is easily to receive the following interesting theorem on the above GDP and the GLDP.

<u>Theorem 10.</u> The GDP and the GLDP with respect to the set of "almost all" global functions $\tau^{(n)}$ in alhabet $A=\{0,1,2,\dots,a-1\}$(a - composite integer), whose local functions $\sigma^{(n)}$ has polynomial representation in the form (3), are equivalent and decidable.

Thus, having a number of results on the problem of decidability of the GDP/GLDP, we cannot spread this achievement on the general case of d-HS, so far. The further investigation on the GDP would be extremely desirable.

The question of the investigation of algorithmical properties of global maps $\tau^{(n)}: \overset{\infty}{C}_A \rightarrow \overset{\infty}{C}_A$ for d-HS($d \geqslant 1$) presents considerable theoretical interest. In connection with this theme the following question arises: Is it decidable whether an arbitrary global map $\tau^{(n)}: \overset{\infty}{C}_A \rightarrow \overset{\infty}{C}_A$ is closed(Closed problem)? For 1-HS Aladyev [10] received the positive answer on this question. This result can be spread on the case d-HS for $d \geqslant 2$.

<u>Theorem 11.</u> The closed problem for d-dimensional($d \geqslant 1$) global maps $\tau^{(n)}: \overset{\infty}{C}_A \rightarrow \overset{\infty}{C}_A$ is decidable.

Aladyev and others [1,10] investigated the problem of interconnection of the minimal size of NCF and MEC in d-HS. However, no one has been able, as yet, to receive a satisfactory solution of this problem. The following result elucidate the reason of such phenomenon.

<u>Theorem 12.</u> It is impossibly, in general, to receive a satisfactory numerical estimation of the minimal size of NCF in d-HS($d \geqslant 1$) depending on the minimal size of MEC, and vice versa.

This result explain the failure of all previous endeavours on this direction. At the same time we receive the answer on Aladyev's problem 5 [10] about the dependence between the minimal size of NCF and MEC in d-HS($d \geqslant 1$). The class of d-HS which has universal reproducing capability in the Moore's sense is enough exceptional in many respect. The next theorem to a certain extent define such class of d-HS($d \geqslant 1$).

<u>Theorem 13.</u> If d-HS($d \geqslant 1$) possesses the universal reproduction in the Moore's sense then for it there exist NCF-1 without NCF. The inverse assertion is false, in general.

On the basis of theorem 13 can be solved the following extremely interesting problem: Can a d-HS($d \geqslant 1$) double any finite CF $c \in \overline{C}_A$? The next result gives answer for case d-HS.

<u>Theorem 14.</u> There exists no d-HS with alphabet A which can double the arbitrary d-dimensional CF $c \in \overline{C}_A$ ($d \geqslant 1$).

In Aladyev [2] the following problem was formulated: Is it decidable whether an arbitrary infinite set $GS \subset \overline{C}_A$ is an $L(\tau_n)$-language? The decisive algorithm is called <u>constructive</u> if it in the case of positive answer give τ_n-grammars themselves which generate $L(\tau_n)$-language GS. In the light of this definition we present now the solution of the more common problem, actually.

<u>Theorem 15.</u> There exists no the constructive algorithm for solution of the problem: Is it decidable whether an arbitrary infinite set GS from $\overline{C}_A$ is an $L(\tau_n)$-language.

In the process of investigation of the GDP by the group methods, Aladyev [10] proved that a semigroup L(a,d) of all d-dimensional maps $\tau^{(n)}: C_A \rightarrow C_A$ can be presented in the form of union of four subsemigroups, which has no finite systems of generators, and a maximum group G(d). At the same place we formulated the Hypothesis 2: G(d) is a single group, i.e. it consists of global functions $\tau^{(n)}$ which carry out identical maps $\tau^{(n)}: C_A \rightarrow C_A$, only. The further investigations show that question with group G(d) is open to a certain extent up to this point. We attempted the detailed investigation of binary 1-HS with the purpose of discovering of an one-one maps $\tau^{(n)}: C_A \rightarrow C_A$, which differ from identical ones. The attempted investigation proved to be a success. The next theorem present the best received result in this direction.

<u>Theorem 16.</u> For any integer $n \geqslant 3$ there exist at any rate $2^{n-1}-n$ binary 1-dimensional functions $\tau^{(n)}$, which possess the following properties, simultaneously:

1. $\tau^{(n)}$ has no NCF and NCF-1;
2. each CF $c \in \overline{C}_A$ is periodical for such global functions;
3. map $\tau^{(n)}: \overset{\infty}{C}_A \rightarrow \overset{\infty}{C}_A$ is not one-one mapping;
4. for function $\tau^{(n)}$ the GDP has negative solution.

This theorem is essential generalization of lemmas 7,9 from our work [10] but it give not exhaustive solution of the problem for the case of binary 1-dimensional global functions, even. Whereas, for the case of non-binary maps $\tau^{(n)}$ our Hypothesis 2 [10] to be wrong, i.e. group G(d) contains nontrivial identical one-one maps. This affirmation is based on the following result.

<u>Theorem 17.</u> A semigroup L(a,1)($a \geqslant 3$) of all 1-dimensional maps $\tau^{(n)}: C_A \rightarrow C_A$ can be presented in the form of union of four subsemigroups, which has no finite systems of generators, and a maximum group G(1), which is union of subgroup T of all identical maps $\tau_o^{(n)}$ ($n > 2$),

and symmetrical subgroup P(a) of periodical maps(global functions) $\tau^{(n)}$ $(n \geq 2)$ with the finite system P(a,2) of generators and correlation $\tau^{(n)(a-1)!} = \tau_0^{(2)}$, and, possibly, subgroup of one-one maps, which differ from above-mentioned ones.

Theorem 17 shows that further work on this problem is badly needed. The complexity is one of the most intriguing and vague concepts in the most cases. At present, we know three approaches to the definition of complexity of the finite objects: combinatorical, probabilistic and algorithmical. For the last case N. Kolmogorov defined the relative complexity of some object G(comparatively of object S) by the minimum length of Turing machine's program of deriving of G from S. Our approach can be also called algorithmical but it differs from Kolmogorov's one [2,3,10]. The essence of our concept of complexity consists in the estimation of complexity of growing of arbitrary finite CF from some primitive CF c_p by means of the finite number of global functions from some set T_f. On the basis of introduced concept of complexity A(X) of the finite CF we presented solutions of a number of problems in the HS theory. The relation between the concept of complexity A(X) and the GDP in d-HS was stated. Furthermore, the relation between A(X) and other famous measures of complexity was presented. However, it is known that our concept of complexity is based on the Hypothesis 3[2]. In our work[6] the proof of this Hypothesis was presented. The general result is expressed by the following theorem.

__Theorem 18.__ For any finite alphabet A there exist no the finite sets of CF $c_i \in \overline{C}_A$ and global functions in alphabet A such that

$$\bigcup_i \langle c_i \rangle \left[\tau^{(n_i)} \right] = \overline{C}_A \qquad (i=\overline{1,k})$$

Theorem 18 allows to give the clean mathematical reasons to a number of results, which were presented in our previous works. On the basis of theorem 18 and the concept of complexity of the finite CF in d-HS$(d \geq 1)$ a number of interesting results can be proved.

__Theorem 19.__ Supplement of the finite set of $L(\widehat{\tau}_n)$-languages cannot be the language of the same type.

This theorem proves the truth of our Hypothesis 4[2], also. In our work[2] was proved that for d-HS without NCF, but with the set W of NCF-1 there exists no the finite set of CF $c_i \in \overline{C}_A$ such that

$$\bigcup_i \langle c_i \rangle \left[\tau^{(n)} \right] = \overline{C}_A \setminus W$$

Now we shall present essentially more general and very strong result, which gives answer on a number of questions formulated in our previous works [1-5,10].

<u>Theorem 20.</u> Let $\tau^{(n)}$ be an arbitrary global function in alphabet A (a - prime), which has the set W of NCF and, possibly, NCF-1. Then there exists no the finite set of CF $c_i \in \overline{C}_A$ and global functions in the alphabet A such that

$$\bigcup_i \langle c_i \rangle \left[\tau^{(n_i)}\right] = \overline{C}_A \setminus W \quad \text{or} \quad \bigcup_i \langle c_i \rangle \left[\tau^{(n_i)}\right] = W \quad (i=\overline{1,k})$$

For the case of composite integer a take place the second correlation.

From this theorem we have a very interesting consequence: sets W and $\overline{C}_A \setminus W$ (W is a set of NCF and, possibly, NCF-1) in the case of prime a cannot be generated by means of the finite sets of CF $c_i \in \overline{C}_A$ and the global functions $\tau^{(n_i)}$ $(i=\overline{1,k})$ in alphabet A regardless of global function $\tau^{(n)}$ respect to which the nonconstructibility is considered. Furthermore, from the result follows that d-HS are finitely non-axiomatized formal parallel systems on the set $\overline{C}_A$. Thus, each set of nonconstructible CF (NCF or NCF-1) with respect to the completeness problem possesses the same immunity with the set $\overline{C}_A$.

In our monograph [2] in connection with the investigation of complexity problem of the finite CF in d-HS the following question was formulated: Can the set of CF of each level of complexity be finite? The next theorem to a certain extent clarifies the gist of the matter.

<u>Theorem 21.</u> There exists the infinite number of basic sets T_f of global functions $\tau^{(n_i)}$ $(i=\overline{1,k})$ with respect to which there exist the infinite sets of the finite CF of the same complexity.

This theorem gives answers on a number of questions presented in Aladyev [2,10]. However, for the complete solution it is necessary in detail to investigate global functions, which form the minimal basic set T_f. We have defined the <u>minimal</u> basic set as a set contained a very insignificant number of global functions. In this direction we have a number of the interesting results.

<u>Theorem 22.</u> There exists a minimal basic set T_f which contains only four 1-dimensional binary global functions. At any rate a function $\tau^{(n)}$ from the set T_f possesses NCF-1, to say the least.

<u>Theorem 23.</u> With respect to the minimal basic set T_f of 1-dimensional binary global functions, there exist infinite sets of the finite CF of the same complexity.

<u>Theorem 24.</u> There exist the minimal basic sets T_f of the binary global functions with respect to which take place the infinite sets of

binary functions $\tau^{(n_i)}$ and binary CF $c_i \in \overline{C}_A$ such that sequences $\langle c_i \rangle [\tau^{(n_i)}]$ contain the binary CF of any given complexity. There exists no the finite basic set T_f of binary global functions with respect to which each sequence $\langle c_o \rangle [\tau^{(n)}] (c_o \in \overline{C}_A)$ contains binary CF of the limited complexity, only.

Theorem 24 gives answer both on our question [10] and forms the basis of the following extremely interesting result. Above we have noted the difference between concepts of complexity A(X) and K(X)(according to Kolmogorov) of the finite objects. The next theorem establishes the difference between the concepts K(X) and A(X).

Theorem 25. There exists the difference of principle with respect to the concepts of complexity K(X) and A(X) between the generative possibilities of the infinite automata MT and 1-HS, which form a base for the above-mentioned concepts of complexity of the finite objects.

This theorem allows to elucidate the difference between of a number of Kolmogorov's and our results on the complexity of the finite objects. We [6] essentially used for the proofs of theorems 20-24 the concept of the minimal basic set T_f and some properties of global functions of T_f; ibid the detailed properties of such minimal basic sets T_f were presented.

Up to now, we considered two concepts of nonconstructibility in d-HS(NCF and NCF-1), only. With the purpose to embrace all possibilities in the problem, we introduced new type of nonconstructibility (NCF-2) in d-HS(d $\geqslant$1) [6].

Definition 4. CF $c \in \overline{C}_A$ is called NCF-2 for global function $\tau^{(n)}$ iff there does not exist CF $\hat{c} \in \overset{\infty}{C}_A$ such that $\hat{c}\,\tau^{(n)}=c$ and there exists CF $c' \in \overline{C}_A$ such that $c'\,\tau^{(n)}=c$.

It is easy to verify that such nonconstructible CF there exist for d-HS(d $\geqslant$1). The next diagram illustrates the essence of all three typies of nonconstructibility in d-HS(d $\geqslant$1).

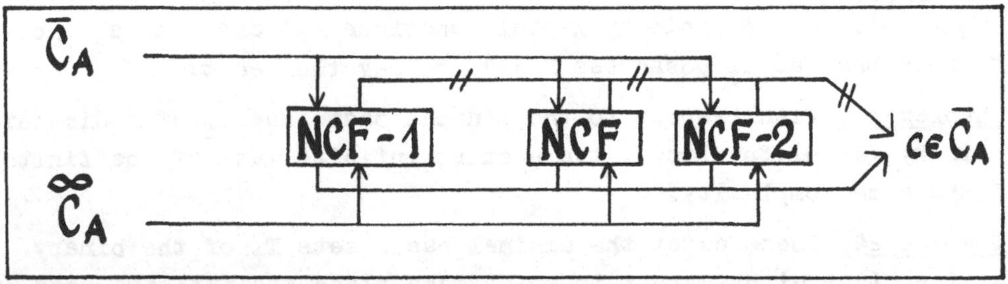

The interconnection of all typies of nonconstructibility in d-HS express the following general result.

Theorem 26. Each d-HS($d \geqslant 1$) simultaneously has typies of nonconsttibility according to the followign table

n/n	NCF	NCF-1	NCF-2	Possibility
1	+	+	+	there exists
2	+	+	-	-//-
3	+	-	+	-//-
4	-	+	+	is absent
5	+	-	-	there exists
6	-	+	-	-//-
7	-	-	+	-//-
8	-	-	-	is absent

The nonempty sets of NCF, NCF-1 and NCF-2 in d-HS($d \geqslant 1$) is infinite, always.

The following theorem gives a criterion of the existence of NCF-2 in 1-HS without NCF.

Theorem 27. 1-dimensional global function $\tau^{(n)}$ without NCF has a NCF-2 iff the corresponding map $\tau^{(n)}: \overset{\infty}{C}_A \to \overset{\infty}{C}_A$ is closed.

This criterion is opposite, in a way, to our criterion of the existence of NCF-1 in 1-HS without NCF. From criteria of the existence of NCF-1 and NCF-2 in 1-HS without NCF the following result can be easily received.

Theorem 28. If 1-dimensional mapping $\tau^{(n)}: \overset{\infty}{C}_A \to \overset{\infty}{C}_A$ is closed (is not closed) then the corresponding global function $\tau^{(n)}$ without NCF possesses NCF-2(NCF-1).

From theorem 26 and algorithmical decidability of the problems of the existence of NCF and NCF-1 in 1-HS the following theorem can be proved.

Theorem 29. The problem of the existence of an arbitrary set of NCF, NCF-1 and NCF-2 in 1-HS is decidable.

It is hardly too much to say, that detailed investigation of the concept of mutually erasable CF(MEC) in d-HS present undoubted interest. This investigations will allow to clarify many dynamic properties of d-HS. Similar work we began in our previous books [1,2,10]; now we introduce the new concept of erasability in d-HS.

Definition 5. Two CR $c_1, c_2 \in C_A$ form for global function $\tau^{(n)}$ a pair of the MEC-1 iff take place the following correlation

$$c_1 \tau^{(n)} = c_2 \tau^{(n)} = c \in \overline{C}_A$$

The given generalization of the concept of erasability is directly linked with the nonconstructibility problem in d-HS. In view of definition 5 the following result can be proved.

Theorem 30. 1-dimensional global function $\tau^{(n)}$ possesses NCF or/and NCF-1 iff for it there exists at least a pair of MEC-1.

This result is the essential generalization of the well-known Moore-Myhill's criterion of the existence of NCF in the 1-HS. The next theorem presents a kind of upper boundary for the existence of typies nonconstructibility in d-HS($d \geqslant 1$).

Theorem 31. Let NCF0, NCF1, NCF2 be sets of all NCF, NCF-1 and NCF-2 with respect to some global function $\tau^{(n)}$, accordingly. Then for each d-dimensional($d \geqslant 1$) global function $\tau^{(n)}$ take place the following correlations:

$$\mathrm{NCF0} \subset \overline{C}_A \ ; \ \mathrm{NCF1} \subset \overline{C}_A \quad \text{and} \quad \mathrm{NCF0} \cup \mathrm{NCF1} \subset \overline{C}_A$$

There exist global functions for which take place the correlation $\mathrm{NCF2} = \overline{C}_A$.

This result gives one of argument in favour of the essential difference between typies of nonconstructibility NCF and NCF-1, on the one hand, and NCF-2, on the other hand. Using now the concept of NCF-2 and proofs of theorems 20 and 26, we can to generalize the theorem 20 on the case of NCF-2.

Theorem 32. Let $\tau^{(n)}$ be an arbitrary global function in alphabet A(a - prime) having set G of NCF-2. Then there does not exist set of CF $c_i \in \overline{C}_A$ and global functions in the same alphabet such that

$$\bigcup_i \langle c_i \rangle \left[\tau_i^{(n_i)} \right] = G \qquad (i=\overline{1,k})$$

On the basis of new results on nonconstructibility in our work[6] the following theorem may be drawn.

Theorem 33. d-dimensional($d \geqslant 1$) global function $\tau^{(n)}$ without NCF possesses NCF-1 iff the corresponding mapping $\tau^{(n)}: \overset{\infty}{C}_A \rightarrow \overset{\infty}{C}_A$ is not closed, i.e. there exists CF $\hat{c} \in \overset{\infty}{C}_A$ such that take place the following correlation $\hat{c}\tau^{(n)} = \overline{0}$.

This theorem gives answer both on a number of questions from our book[2] and our problem 1[10]. Furthermore, it can be used for generalization of a number of the above-mentioned results on nonconstructibility in d-HS($d \geqslant 1$). The following theorem presents a number of results, which are linked with the generalization of the concepts of esazability in homogeneous structures.

<u>Theorem 34.</u> d-dimensional(d$\geqslant$1) global function without NCF possesses NCF-2 iff the corresponding mapping $\tau^{(n)}: \overset{\infty}{C}_A \rightarrow \overset{\infty}{C}_A$ is closed; if mapping $\tau^{(n)}: \overset{\infty}{C}_A \rightarrow \overset{\infty}{C}_A$ is closed(is not closed) then global function $\tau^{(n)}$ without NCF possesses NCF-2(NCF-1). d-dimensional(d$\geqslant$1) function $\tau^{(n)}$ possesses NCF or/and NCF-1 iff for it there exist MEC-1. The problems of the existence of NCF-1 and NCF-2 in d-HS(d$\geqslant$1) without NCF are decidable. If for d-dimensional(d$\geqslant$1) global function $\tau^{(n)}$ there does not exist MEC-1 then for it there exist NCF-2; the inverse affirmation to be wrong, in general.

Theorem 34 essentially generalizes the well-known Moore-Myhill's criterion of the existence of NCF in d-HS(d$\geqslant$1).

In spite of simplicity of the classical concept of the d-HS, the dynamics of d-HS is enough difficult for investigations by theoretical methods. For this reason, for investigation of the d-HS the different computer simulation programs were created [1,8,9,11,13].

By means of such computer modelling a number of interesting results in the HS theory was obtained. For example, in work [11] we presented a computer simulation system in BASIC language for personal computer ISKRA 226, which allows to model interesting subclass of 2-HS - HS with refractority(2-HSR). Such structures present undoubted interest for a number of applications [12]. With help of computer modelling of 2-HSR a number of dynamic properties of the structures was obtained.

However, this approach has essential limitations. Indeed, on the basis of the optimal algorithms of modelling we stated that time T of modelling of one step of some d-HS is directly proportional to quantity K^d, i.e. $T=f\cdot K^d$, where K is size of d-dimensional hypercube edge and f is almost-constant numerical function dependent on the global transition function of d-HS.

Consequently, (d-HS) - like problems are NP-complete ones. Therefore the problems are difficult for modelling on computers in real time: the deep of analysis of d-HS dynamics is limited by the computer productivity, on the whole.

Thus, similar parallel dynamic cellular systems to the best advantage are exactly modelled on the computing cellular structures, for which the d-HS is a formal parallel model [11-13].

At the end of the paper we shall present solutions of a number of well-known mathematical problems from combinatorics and number theory. These problems once again corroborate the effectiveness of methods of the HS theory for the investigations of the mathematical problems.

In the well-known journal "Scientific American" for March 1984 by Haies was presented the unsolved problem "Flights and falls of numbers-hailstones", the essence of which can be formulated as follows.

Let $p_o=n$ be initial number, where $n>0$ is arbitrary integer. The subsequent integers are generated in the following recurrent rule:

$$p_i = \begin{cases} p_{i-1}/2 & \text{, if } p_{i-1} \text{ is even number} \\ 3p_{i-1} & \text{, if } p_{i-1} \text{ is odd number} \end{cases}$$

$$p_o=n \qquad (i=1,2,3,\dots)$$

Numbers p_i form the numerical sequence $SG(p_o)=\{p_i\}$ $(i=0,1,2,\dots)$. The following general question can be formulated: Is it possible to state the algorithm of behaviour of $SG(p_o)$-sequence elements(numbers-hailstones) for each integer $p_o>0$?

In this connection we have recently investigated this problem combining some theoretical methods and numerical experiments on the personal computer ISKRA 226 [8,11]. Such approach allows to establish the behaviour of $SG(p_o)$-sequence for any initial integer $p_o>0$. In brief outline the essence of such approach comes to the following.

For numerical experiments with sequence $SG(p_o)$ was worked out the mathematical program for personal computer(PC) ISKRA 226 in BASIC-language. This program essentially use some quik parallel algorithms of 1-HS. As a result the computation time of the numerical experiments with $SG(p_o)$-sequences decreases to a large degree. The numerical experiments on the PC ISKRA 226 allow to prove that any $SG(p_o)$-sequence contains element $p_i=4$ for $p_o \leqslant 2000000$; $i=i(p_o)$. On the other hand, theoretical methods allow to prove that any $SG(p_o)$-sequence contains some element $p_k \leqslant 2000000$. On the basis of the above-mentioned results the following interesting theorem can be formulated.

<u>Theorem 35.</u> For any integer $p_o>0$ there exists integer $m=m(p_o)>0$ such that element $m=m(p_o)$ in the $SG(p_o)$-sequence is equal to 4, i.e. each $SG(p_o)$-sequence is periodical with period $l=3$, leading with element $m=m(p_o)$ (integer $p_o>0$).

This theorem gives complete answer on the above-mentioned question. To our knowledge this result is the best of its kind.

S. Ulam [1] has attempted to define heuristic studies of the growth in 1-dimensional case on the basis of so-called "unique sum sequences" (USS). Unfortunately, even here it is not easy to establish properties of these USS. By Aladyev and others [1,2,10] theoretical and experimental investigations of a modification of the USS were fulfilled. We investigated such 1-dimensional model of growth by means of 2-HS and computer modelling. Then, Aladyev [8,11] worked out the self-organizing program in BASIC-language for PC ISKRA 226 (WANG 2200), which allows to carry out enough wide experiments with the USS.

Let N be set of all positive integers. Define binary operation w as w: X+Y $\longrightarrow$ P (X,Y,P $\in$ N) on the set N. Elements P form a set N' $\subset$ N. We shall consider only two typies of binary operation w defined on the set N:

(1) w_1: starting with the integers a and b(a < b) we construct new ones in sequence by considering sums of two previously defined integers, but not including in our collection those integers which can be obtained as a sum of previous ones in more than one way(obligatory condition: we never add an integer to itself; in addition take part the very right elements of the previous sections of the USS). Such sequences are denoted by USS1(a,b);

(2) w_2: by analogy with w_1, but on condition that the second obligatory condition is omitted. Such sequences are denoted by USS2(a,b).

The elements a_i and a_{i+1} of the USSk(a,b)(k=1,2) are called the <u>twins</u> if $a_{i+1} - a_i = p(a,b)$. The set of all twins for the USSk(a,b) (k=1,2) is denoted by B(p). Both modifications of the USS(a,b) has a number of interesting interpretations. In this direction, using computer modelling and theoretical results in a class of 2-HS, the following interesting theorem can be formulated.

<u>Theorem 36.</u> Each USS2(a,b) has the infinite set of twins at least a type B(a), B(b) or B(a+b). The USS1(a,2a) has the infinite set B(2a); the density of the USS1(a,2a) with respect to the set N is equal to 0; for the USS1(a,2a) there exists formula $a_k=f(k,a)$ which allows to expresses elements a_k of the sequence through variables a and k. The USS1(1,b) has the infinite sets B(b), B(b+1) for each integer b $\geqslant$ 3; elements a_k of such sequences are expressed by formulas $a_k=f_3(k,b)$ (b=3), $a_k=f_4(k,b)$ (b=4) and $a_k=f_5(k,b)$ (b $\geqslant$ 5). If a > 1 and b/a-[b/a] > 0 then in the USS1(a,b) all elements a_k of sequence are expressed by the formulae $a_k=b+(k-2)a$ (k=3,4,5,...); the set B(b) in such sequences USS1(a,b) is infinite.

To our knowledge this result is the best of its kind.

Now we shall present a solution of well-known Steinhays's problem which can be formulated as follows. Let $c_t=p(1,1)\ ...\ p(1,t)$ be the first string of length t of binary elements $p(1,i)(i=\overline{1,t})$ and number $t \in \{3+4k$ or $4+4k;\ k=0,1,2,\ldots\}$. The elements of the k-th string of length t-k+1 are derived in connection with the following recurrent rule:

$$p(k,i) = p(k-1,i) + p(k-1,i+1) + 1 \pmod 2$$
$$(i=\overline{1,t-k+1};\ k=\overline{2,t})$$

As a result, we have a triangular figure F_t which consists of symbols 0 and 1. The string c_t is called a solution of Steinhays's problem for the value t(S(t)-problem) if from it can be derived the figure F_t which contains the same number $t(t+1)/4$ of symbols 0 and 1. We start from some remarks and definitions to present S(t)-problem's solutions.

Let S(t) be the set of all kinds solutions of S(t)-problem. It is easily verified that S(3)={000, 011, 101, 110} and S(4)={0011, 0101, 1010, 1011, 1100, 1101}; these two sets are called the basic sets. Solution S(t) is called derivative (D(t), if it can be presented in the form of concatenation $S(t)=S(t_1)S(t_2)\ \ldots\ S(t_n)$ of solutions $S(t_i)$ with $t_i < t,\ \sum t_i = t\ (i=\overline{1,n})$. A derivative solution D(t) is called basic (B(t)) if in its D(t)-representations $S(t_i) \in S(3) \cup S(4)$ for $i=\overline{1,n}$.

For the purpose of modelling of the process of generation of the above-mentioned figures F_t, we defined a special 2-HS. The detailed analysis of such 2-HS, which uses the profound properties of the global functions $\tau^{(4)}$, shows that for each permitted value $t \geqslant 3$ S(t) - problem has positive solutions. At the same time, a series of the interesting properties of S(t)-problem's solutions can be drawn. On the basis of such analysis and computer modelling on the personal computer ISKRA 226 Aladyev[6-8,11] proved the following general result.

Theorem 37. Let S(t), D(t) and B(t) be the sets of all solutions, derivative and basic solutions of the S(t)-problem, accordingly. Then for any permitted value $t \geqslant 11$ take place the following correlations:

$$\#\ S(t) > \#\ D(t) > \#\ B(t) > t.$$

For any permitted value t take place the following correlations:

$$\#\ S(t) \gg 2^{t-r(t)}, \text{ where } r(t) \leqslant [t/2], \text{ and}$$

$$\#\ B(t) \geqslant \begin{cases} 2^{3k-2}, & \text{if } t \in \{3+4k\} \\ 2^{3k}, & \text{if } t \in \{4+4k\} \end{cases} \quad (k=1,2,3,\ldots)$$

where $\#\ U$ denotes the cardinality of the set U. Similar results take place for case of derivative solutions, also.

Thus, theorem 37 gives solution of the S(t)-problem formulated by Steinhays for mathematicians (professionals and amateurs) more 25 years ago. It is important to observe, too, that S(t)-problem can be generalized and results of theorem 37 can be generalized accordingly. Furthermore, we received a number of more specific results on the S(t)-problem, which can be found in Aladyev[6-8,11].

At last, we can use the homogeneous cellular space of d-HS independently. Indeed, the principle of homogeneous dividing of space E^n combined with analytical methods can be productively used for solving a number of problems. Thus, this approach can be used for investigations of properties of solutions of some classes of equations in whole numbers. For example, the well known Big Fermat's Problem (BFP) reads:

there exists no solutions of equation

$$X^n + Y^n = Z^n \qquad n > 2 \tag{4}$$

in positive whole numbers. At present, the full solution of the BFP is absent. But using the above mentioned approach we obtain an interesting property of equation (4):

For enough large integers n triplets in whole numbers

$$\langle x, y, z\rangle \quad (x, y > 0;\ 0 < z \leqslant [n/\ln 2] + 1)$$

cannot be solutions of equation (4). Thus, the idea of homogeneous cellular space is very productive, independently.

I hope that this work will help to clear up some general aspects of the mathematical theory of HS and its applications as well as giving information about the latest our results to scientists working on this topic of the modern cybernetics.

4. CONCLUDING REMARKS

In conclusion of the present discussion of new results on the HS theory I should like once more to note about necessity of the very wide popularization of the theory and their possibilities in computer science and modelling for the purpose of attracting the largest number of researches in the different areas to investigations on the HS theory and their applications in the computer systems of new generations. It is important direction for the further development of the HS theory, also! Indeed, many aspects of the HS theory demand active participation of scientists of the different areas: pure and applied mathematics, physics, theoretical and mathematical biology, parallel programming, enginnering and many others.

On the other hand, the HS theory can exercise considerable influence on a number of areas. The appearance of great many new problems in the theory of HS is waited for employment of HS for modelling in a new areas. It is hardly too much to say that the HS theory is in the making, and further work on this perspective theme is badly needed.

REFERENCES

1. Aladyev V.: To Theory of Homogeneous Structures. Estonian Academic Press. Tallinn 1972, 259 p.
2. Aladyev V.: Mathematical Theory of Homogeneous Structures and Their Applications. Valgus Press. Tallinn 1980, 268 p.
3. Aladyev V.: New results in the theory of homogeneous structures. Informatik-Skripten 8, Braunschweig 1984, 3-15.
4. Aladyev V.: A few results in homogeneous structures. Parallel Processing by Cellular Automata. PARCELLA-84. Akademie-Verlag. Berlin 1985, 3-16.
5. Aladyev V.: New results in the theory of homogeneous structures. MTA. Szamitastechn. es autom. kut. intez. tanul., no. 158(1984), 3-14.
6. Aladyev V.: Solutions of a Number of Problems in the Theory of Homogeneous Structures. TR-040684, P/A "Silikaat". Tallinn 1985, 60 p.
7. Aladyev V.: Recent Results on the Theory of Homogeneous Structures. TR-061285, P/A "Silikaat". Tallinn 1985, 30 p.
8. Aladyev V.: Architecture and Software of Personal Computer ISKRA 226. SKB MPSM ESSR. Tallinn 1986, 70 p.
9. Parallel Processing and Parallel Algorithms(Ed. by V. Aladyev). Valgus Press. Tallinn 1981, 298 p.
10. Parallel Processing Systems(Ed. by V. Aladyev). Valgus Press. Tallin 1983, 370 p.
11. Aladyev V. et al.: Programming in Personal Computer ISKRA 226. Technika. Kiev 1987, 250 p.
12. Aladyev V.: Homogeneous structures in modelling. Proc. of the 6-th Intern. Conf. on Mathem. Modelling(1987), St.-Louis, USA.
13. Aladyev V.: Theoretical and Applied Aspects of Homogeneous Structures, in: Methods of Digital Information Processing. Tallinn 1987

A NOTE ON THE RATIO FUNCTION IN DOL SYSTEMS (Extended Abstract)

Mária Kráľová
Institute of Computer Science, Comenius University
842 43 Bratislava, Czechoslovakia

I. INTRODUCTION

L systems have been designed as models of development in multicellular organisms. One of the most thoroughly investigated classes of L systems are the so called DOL systems (deterministic informationless Lindenmayer systems), which have been important for mathematical and biological theories such as the theory of growth functions (first introduced in [9]).

Growth functions are the functions on L systems with a biological origin. In addition to it, the letter occurrence function (see e.g. [10]) and the ratio function introduced in [5] are biological motivated special functions on L systems. The ratio function corresponds to such notions as the mitotic index or FLM curve (Fraction Labelled Mitosis curve) are.

In [5] the behaviour of the ratio function of a DOL system is studied according to structural properties of the given DOL system. In the present paper we continue the study of the properties of the ratio function for the case, when it is determined by an expanding letter with the index of expansion $i \geq 1$.

The paper is divided into four parts. In the part II the basic notions and notations are given. In the part III the index of expansion for an expanding letter is introduced and studied. There are shown properties of the levels generated by expanding letters, too. Using this results the theorem on the ratio function determined by an expanding letter with the index of expansion $i \geq 1$ is formulated and proved in last part.

II. BASIC NOTIONS AND NOTATIONS

In this section we recall briefly definitions of L systems to be considered in the paper. Doing this we assume that the reader is familiar with basic notions concerning formal languages. The terminology and the notations used are mostly those of Vitányi in [10]. Perhaps only the following points require an explanation:

$\#_a v$ denotes the number of all occurrences of a in the string v ;
W^* denotes the set of all words (finite strings) over the set W,
ε denotes the empty word,
$W^+ = W^* - \{\varepsilon\}$,
Z^+ denotes the set of nonnegative integers $\{0,1,2,\ldots\}$,
N denotes the set of natural numbers $\{1,2,\ldots\}$.

Definition 1. A **DOL system** (deterministic informationless Lindenmayer system) is an ordered triple $H=(W,h,w)$, where W is a finite nonempty set (the **alphabet** of the system), $h: W^* \to W^*$ is a homomorphism determining the **production rules** and $w \in W^*$ is an initial word (the **axiom** of the system).

Next we define

$$h^0(b) = b$$
$$h^t(b) = h(h^{t-1}(b))$$

for any $b \in W$ and $t \in N$.

Definition 2. Let $H=(W,h,w)$ be a DOL system, let $w' = x_1 x_2 \ldots x_n$, where $x_i \in W$ for $i=1,2,\ldots n$, let $w = y_1 x_1 x_2 \ldots x_n y_2$, where $y_1, y_2 \in W^*$. Then w' is called the **subaxiom** of the axiom w.

Definition 3. An ordered quadruple $\overline{H}=(W,h,w,w')$ is called the **DOL system with the subaxiom**, if (W,h,w) is a DOL system and w' is a subaxiom of the axiom w.

Definition 4. Let $H=(W,h,w)$ be a DOL system. A letter $a \in W$ is called **mortal** $(a \in M)$ if $h^t(a) = \varepsilon$ for some t;
b-mortal for $b \in W$ $(a \in b\text{-}M)$ if there is $n \in N$ that $\#_b h^t(a) = 0$ for all $t \geq n$;
recursive $(a \in R)$ if $h^t(a) \in W^*\{a\}W^*$ for some $t \in N$;
monorecursive $(a \in MR)$ if $h^t(a) \in M^*\{a\}M^*$ for some $t \in N$;
expanding $(a \in E)$ if $h^t(a) \in W^*\{a\}W^*\{a\}W^*$ for some $t \in N$;
accessible from a string $v \in W^*$ $(a \in U(v))$ if $\#_a h^t(v) \neq 0$ for some $t \in N$.

We define an equivalence relation $\equiv$ on W by $a \equiv b$ if $a \in U(b)$ and $b \in U(a)$. Hence $\equiv$ induces a partition of W in equivalence classes

$$[a] = \{b \in W;\ b \equiv a\}$$

and

$$W/_{\equiv} = \{[a];\ a \in W\}.$$

The equivalence class [a] is called the **level** of DOL system generated by a.

<u>Definition 5.</u> The level [a] of the DOL system H generated by a is said to be **monorecursive**, **expanding** iff the letter a is monorecursive, expanding, respectively.

III. THE INDEX OF EXPANSION

In the paper [5] the notion of the index of monorecursivity and expansion is introduced as follows:

<u>Definition 6.</u> Let H=(W,h,w) be a DOL system. A letter $a \in W$ is called **monorecursive with the index of monorecursivity** i ($a \in MR^{(i)}$), **expanding with the index of expansion** i ($a \in E^{(i)}$) if i is the smallest number for which the condition of monorecursivity, expansion, respectively, is satisfied.

<u>Proposition 7.</u> [4] Let H=(W,h,w) be a DOL system and $a, b \in W$, $b \in [a]$. Let P be one of the sets MR, E. Then $a \in P$ iff $b \in P$.

It is clear from this proposition that any letter of the monorecursive (expanding) level is monorecursive (expanding). But this proposition says nothing about the index of monorecursivity or expansion.

<u>Proposition 8.</u> Let [a] be a monorecursive level of a DOL system H=(W,h,w) and let $a \in MR^{(i)}$. Then every $b \in [a]$ is a monorecursive letter with the index of monorecursivity i.

However, as regards the index of expansion of the single letters in the same expanding level, it can have different values for different letters. To illustrate this fact we give two very simple examples.

<u>Example 1.</u> Let us consider a DOL system H=(W,h,w), where W = {a,b}, h(a) = b, h(b) = aa. Then the production trees (similar to the production trees of context free grammars) for the letter a, b have the form

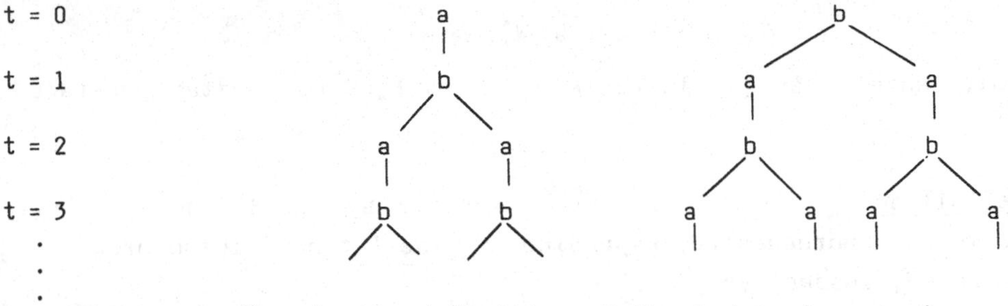

Then according to the definition of the index of expansion we have $a \in E^{(2)}$, $b \in E^{(2)}$.

<u>Example 2.</u> Let a DOL system D=(W,h,w) be given as follows W = {a,b}, h(a) = ab, h(b) = a. Derivations starting with the letters of the alphabet W give the following sequences of strings

a, ab, aba, abaab, abaababa, ...
b, a, ab, aba, abaab, ...

Evidently $a \in E^{(2)}$, $b \in E^{(4)}$, i.e. i = 2 for the letter a and i = 4 for the letter b.

In the next part we shall investigate a special condition securing the same index of expansion for all letters of the same expanding level. We shall define this condition as follows:

Consider a DOL system H=(W,h,w). Let $a \in W$ be an expanding letter . Then we shall say that a letter $b \in W$ **satisfies the condition C1** if for its production rule

$$h(b) = u \tag{1}$$

it holds: there is only one letter $c \in [a]$ such that $u \in (a\text{-}M \cup \{c\})^{+}$.

Further a relevance of the condition C1 will be shown.

<u>Lemma 9.</u> Let H=(W,h,w) be a DOL system and $a \in W$ be an expanding letter with the index of expansion $i \geq 1$. Let every $b \in [a]$ satisfy the condition C1. Then the level [a] contains exactly i letters.

Proof sketch: First assume i = 1. In this case the assertion of the lemma follows easily from definitions above.

Let $i \geq 1$. The condition C1 implies that the word u (occurring in the right side of the relation (1)) can be expressed in the form

$$x_1 c_s x_2 c_s \dots x_{k_s} c_s x_{k_s+1}, \tag{2}$$

where $x_1, x_2, \dots x_{k_s+1} \in W^*$ consist of a-mortal letters only and $c_s \in [a]$.

We note that any word having the form (2) can be composed of a certain number of more simple words that can be written as

$$v c_s y, \tag{3}$$

$v, y \in (a\text{-}M \cap W)^*$, $c_s \in [a]$. Because c_s is the same letter occurring in each subword of the form (3), it suffices to assume the word u (from the right side of (1)) to be in the form (3).

Since $a \in [a]$ and $a \in E^{(i)}$, $i \geq 1$, there exist words $v_1, v_2, \dots v_i, y_1, \dots y_{i-1} \in (a\text{-}M \cap W)^*$ and letters $c_1, c_2, \dots c_{i-1} \in [a]$ such that $h(a) = v_1 c_1 y_1$, $h(c_1) = v_2 c_2 y_2$, ... $h(c_{i-2}) = v_{i-1} c_{i-1} y_{i-1}$, $h(c_{i-1}) = v_i a y_i$.

It is clear that $c_s \neq a$ for $s = 1, 2, \dots i-1$ and $c_k \neq c_j$ for $k \neq j$ (it follows from the assumption $a \in E^{(i)}$).

<u>Theorem 10.</u> Let $H=(W,h,w)$ be a DOL system and let $a \in W$ be an expanding letter with the index of expansion $i \geq 1$. If every letter $b \in [a]$ satisfies the condition C1, then the level [a] contains expanding letters with the index of expansion exactly i, only.

IV. RATIO FUNCTIONS

To study ratio functions of DOL systems it is sufficient to consider DOL systems reduced in such a way that all letters in the alphabet are accessible from the axiom only, i.e. for every letter $b \in W$ there is a number $t \in Z^+$ such that $h^t(w) = xby$, $x, y \in W^*$. For those DOL systems we shall give the characterization of the ratio function determined by an expanding letter with the index of expansion $i \geq 1$ similarly as in the case of the ratio function determined by a monorecursive letter (it was first discussed in [5].

<u>Definition 11.</u> Let $\overline{H}=(W,h,w,w')$ be a DOL system with the subaxiom and $a \in W$. The function $r_a: Z_a \longrightarrow \langle 0,1 \rangle$, where $Z_a = \{k \in Z^+;\ \#_a h^k(w) \neq 0\}$, defined by

$$r_a(t) = \frac{\#_a h^t(w')}{\#_a h^t(w)}$$

is called the **ratio function** of $\overline{H}$ determined by the letter a.

Let us recall assertions of theorems, in which the ratio function is determined by $a \in MR^{(i)}$, $i \geq 1$, and $a \in E^{(1)}$.

Theorem 12. Assume a DOL system $\overline{H}=(W,h,w,w')$ with the subaxiom and let $[a]$ be its monorecursive level with the index of monorecursivity 1. Let every $b \in W - \{a\}$ satisfy one of the conditions C2, C3.

C2: $b \in a\text{-}M$,

C3: $b \notin R$ and $a \in U(b)$.

Then either $Z_a = \emptyset$ or there are numbers $t_0, q \in N$, $p \in Z^+$ such that

$$r_a(t) = \frac{p}{q} \quad \text{for } t \geq t_0.$$

Theorem 13. Let $\overline{H}=(W,h,w,w')$ be a DOL system with the subaxiom and $a \in W$ be an expanding letter with the index of expansion 1. If for every $b \in W - \{a\}$ the condition C3 is fulfilled, thus either $Z_a = \emptyset$ or there exist a rational number $\frac{p}{q} \in \langle 0,1 \rangle$ and $t_0 \in Z^+$ that

$$r_a(t) = \frac{p}{q} \quad \text{for } t \geq t_0.$$

Theorem 14. Let $\overline{H}=(W,h,w,w')$ be a DOL system with the subaxiom, $[a]$ be its monorecursive level with the index of monorecursivity $i \geq 1$. Let one of the previous conditions C2, C3 and C4: $a \in U(b)$ and $b \in MR$ be satisfied for every $b \in W - \{a\}$. Then either $Z_a = \emptyset$ or there is a number $t_0 \in Z^+$ such, that the ratio function $r_a(t)$ is periodic with the period i (the length of its preperiod is equal to t_0).

We turn our attention to the ratio function determined by an expanding letter with the index of expansion $i \geq 1$. The analog of Theorem 14 can be proved.

Theorem 15. Assume a DOL system with the subaxiom and $a \in W$ an expanding letter with the index of expansion $i \geq 1$. Let a satisfy the condition C1. If one of following conditions

1. $a \notin U(b)$,
2. $a \in U(b)$ and $b \notin R$,
3. $b \in [a]$ and b satisfies the condition C1

is fulfilled for every $b \in W - \{a\}$, then either $Z_a = \emptyset$ or there is a $t_0 \in N$ such that $r_a(t)$ is a periodic function with the period i and with the preperiod of the length t_0.

Proof sketch. Because $a \in E^{(t)}$ and a satisfies the condition C1 we can write

$$\#_a h^i(a) \geq 2$$

$$\#_a h^t(a) = 0,$$

where $1 \leq t < i$.

Let us denote

$$\#_a h^i(a) = m.$$

Then it holds clearly

$$\#_a h^t(a) = \begin{cases} m^n & \text{if } t = ni,\ n \in Z^+, \\ 0 & \text{if } t \neq ni,\ n \in Z^+. \end{cases} \qquad (2)$$

To prove that the ratio function of $\overline{H}$ determined by a is a periodic function (with the preperiod of the length t_0) we must prove that it holds

$$r_a(t_0+ni+j) = r_a(t_0+j),$$

where $j = 0,1,\dots i-1$, $n \in Z^+$.

It is easy to see: if $a \notin U(b)$, then $\#_a h^t(b) = 0$ for all $t \in Z^+$. Therefore it suffices to analyse remaining two cases.

Assume

$$B = \{b \in W;\ a \in U(b) \text{ and } b \notin R\}$$

and

$$\text{card } B = s,\ s \in Z^+.$$

Now, construct an oriented graph P of the relation $\triangleright$ that the set of vertices V is given as $V = \{b \in W;\ b \in [a] \text{ or } b \in B\}$. We note that this graph doesn t contain isolated points and $a \triangleright b$ iff $h(a) = xby$ for some $x,y \in W^*$. Let d_k is the length of the path from b_k to a.

Let us define

$$d = \begin{cases} \max_k d_k & k = 1,2,\dots s,\ s \neq 0 \\ 0 & \text{if } s = 0 \text{ (i.e. card } B = 0) \end{cases}$$

Put

$$t_0 = d.$$

Thus

$$\#_a h^{t_0+ni}(b_k) = \#_a h^{t_0}(b_k)m^n$$

for $k = 1,2,\ldots s$, $n \in Z^+$.

Let us assume $b \in [a]$ be such that b satisfies condition C1. By Lemma 9 the level [a] consists of i letters. One of them is the letter a and we shall denote by $c_1, c_2, \ldots c_{i-1}$ the additional letters of this level. We shall suppose further that

$$\#_{c_j} h^j(a) \neq 0 \qquad \text{for } j = 1,2,\ldots i-1.$$

Then Theorem 10 implies immediately

$$\#_a h^{ni}(c_j) = 0 \qquad \text{for } j = 1,2,\ldots i-1,\ n \in Z^+ .$$

Now, we can proceed to the expression of the ratio function determined by a.

If $t_0 = 0$ then

$$r_a(ni) = \frac{\#_a w'}{\#_a w},$$

$$r_a(ni+j) = \frac{\#_{c_{i-j}} w' \#_a h^j(c_{i-j})}{\#_{c_{i-j}} w \#_a h^j(c_{i-j})}.$$

If $t_0 > 0$ then

$$r_a(t_0+ni+j) = \frac{\#_a h^{t_0+j}(a)\#_a w' + \#_a h^{t_0+j}(c_{i-k_j})\#_{c_{i-k_j}} w' + \sum_{b \in B} \#_a h^{t_0+j}(b)\#_b w'}{\#_a h^{t_0+j}(a)\#_a w + \#_a h^{t_0+j}(c_{i-k_j})\#_{c_{i-k_j}} w + \sum_{b \in B} \#_a h^{t_0+j}(b)\#_b w}$$

where $t_0+j = n_j i + k_j$, $k_j < t$ and $c_i = a$, $j = 0,1,\ldots i-1$.

REFERENCES

[1] HERMAN G.T., VITÁNYI P.M.B.: Growth functions associated with biological development, Amer. Math. Monthly 83 (1976) 1-15

[2] HROMKOVIČ J.: Ratio function analysis, Computers and Artificial Intelligence 4 (1985) 2, 137-142

[3] HROMKOVIČ J., KELEMENOVÁ A.: On kinetic models of cell population, Proc. of The 3rd Int. Symp. of System Simulation in Biology and Medicine, Prague, 1982, Microfishe No 735

[4] KELEMENOVÁ A.: Levels in L-systems, Mathematica Slovaca 33 (1983) 1, 87-97

[5] KRÁĽOVÁ M.: Constant ratio-function of Lindenmayer systems, Math. Slovaca 35 (1985) 3, 283-294

[6] LINDENMAYER A.: Mathematical models of cellular interactions in development I, II, Journal of Theoretical Biology, 18 (1968) 280-299, 300-315

[7] LINDENMAYER A., ROZENBERG G.: Automata, Languages, Development, North Holland, Amsterdam 1976

[8] ROZENBERG G., SALOMAA A.: The mathematical Theory of L-systems, Academic Press, New York 1980

[9] SZILARD A.: Growth functions of Lindenmayer systems, Univ. of Western Ontario Computer Science Department Technical Report No 4, London, Canada 1971

[10] VITÁNYI P.M.B.: Lindenmayer Systems: Structure, Languages and Growth functions, Mathematisch Centrum, Amsterdam 1978

MODELS FOR MULTICELLULAR DEVELOPMENT:
CHARACTERIZATION, INFERENCE AND COMPLEXITY OF L-SYSTEMS

A. Lindenmayer
Theoretical Biology Group
University of Utrecht
Padualaan 8
3584 CH Utrecht
The Netherlands

Introduction

L-systems were introduced to model the development of multicellular organisms. Originally they were defined in terms of automata and formal languages [22, 39, 40]. We consider arrays of cells. Each cell can be in one of finitely many states at each discrete time step. Development is modeled by applying substitution (rewriting) rules in parallel to each cell in each time step. Substitutions may program cell divisions or cell death, by adding or erasing cells from the array, or changes in cell states. Neighbourhoods are strictly preserved during these substitutions. The rewriting may be context-free (interactionless development) or context-sensitive (development with interactions). Most of the work is on linear 1-dimensional cellular arrays, but 2-dimensional arrays [73, 74, 78] and branching arrays [19, 25, 39] were also considered. For comprehensive treatments of the mathematical results and later developments in the theory of L-systems see the books [22, 68, 79]. Simulation programs have been written and applied to plant development [3,17,26,29,41] and recently animated films of growing trees and changing landscapes have been produced [2, 62, 76] on the basis of L-systems. Bibliographies of this theory are available in the above mentioned books and in [50].

These systems are different from the cellular automata constructs of von Neumann [59] or from tesselation systems [75, 81] in that the arrays can grow on shrink everywhere instead of only at the margins. They differ, on the other hand, from Chomsky grammars [28] because they require parallel rewriting of all the symbols in the arrays and they do not distinguish between terminal and non-terminal symbols.

More recently a graph-theoretical framework for L-systems has proved to provide a more unified approach to 1-dimensional as well as 2- or 3-dimensional cellular development [7, 8,13a,44, 46, 48, 53]. This graph interpretation is also topological, i.e., it concerns the neighbourhood relationships among cells. To these systems analytical and graphical geometric specifications can be added for lengths, angles, colors, and other properties of cells or their walls and edges. The most useful of these graph-theoretical constructs have been those in which edge labels are the main control elements. In the course of applying these constructs we can make use of many of the results obtained by formal-language-theoretical means.

Three main aspects of L-systems are to be considered: inference, characterization and complexity. Inference questions refer to the problem of finding possible generating systems to an observed sequence of structures. Characterization has to do with the exhibition of mathematical properties of various classes of generating systems, and in particular with proving that it is impossible for a certain class of these systems to generate some sequence of structures. Complexity results are interesting for providing the minimal number of control elements or manipulations which are necessary to generate certain patterns.

Definitions

L-systems are parallel rewriting systems which generate sequences of multi-cellular structures. As mentioned above, two basic types of their definitions have evolved, the first being essentially formal-language-theoretical and the second graph-theoretical. To illustrate these two formalisms, let us consider the development of a multicellular filament such as found in blue-green bacteria and various algae. The symbols a and b represent cytological states of the cells (in this case these have to do with their size and readiness to divide). The arrows indicate cell polarity which plays a role in the orientation of the division, namely the positions in which a and b type cells are produced.

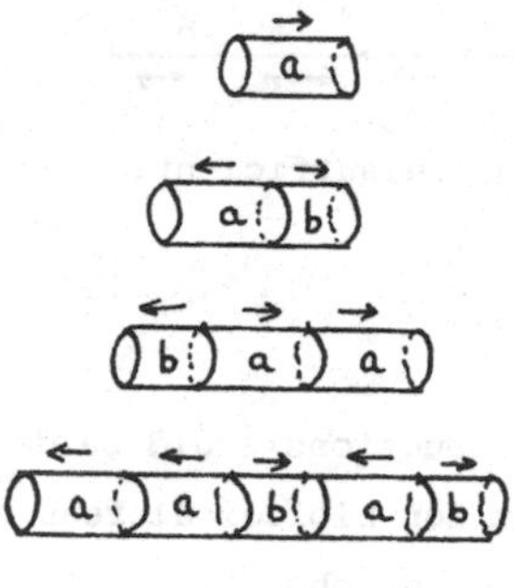

We can combine the 2 cytological states and the 2 polarity states into 4 symbols and obtain the following rewriting rules:

$$\vec{a} \longrightarrow \overleftarrow{a}\ \vec{b} \qquad\qquad \overleftarrow{a} \longrightarrow \overleftarrow{b}\ \vec{a}$$

$$\vec{b} \longrightarrow \vec{a} \qquad\qquad \overleftarrow{b} \longrightarrow \overleftarrow{a}$$

If these rules are applied in parallel to each cell of the filaments, the following sequence of words is obtained as a developmental description:

$$\overrightarrow{a}$$

$$\overleftarrow{a}\ \overrightarrow{b}$$

$$\overleftarrow{b}\ \overrightarrow{a}\ \overrightarrow{a}$$

$$\overleftarrow{a}\ \overleftarrow{a}\ \overrightarrow{b}\ \overleftarrow{a}\ \overrightarrow{b}$$

$$\vdots$$

In the context of formal language theory we speak here of a deterministic parallel rewriting system with context-free rules (a "DOL-system") which generates a single sequence of strings.

The other way of describing this development is by considering rules acting on directed and edge-labeled graphs.

We represent the cylindrical cells of the filament as edges of a linear graph, each edge labeled by a cell state symbol and oriented according to its polarity. Edge production rules are to be applied according to the orientation of each edge, the orientation of a newly generated edge being the same as that of the original if a + sign is attached to its label, and opposite if a - sign is attached to it.

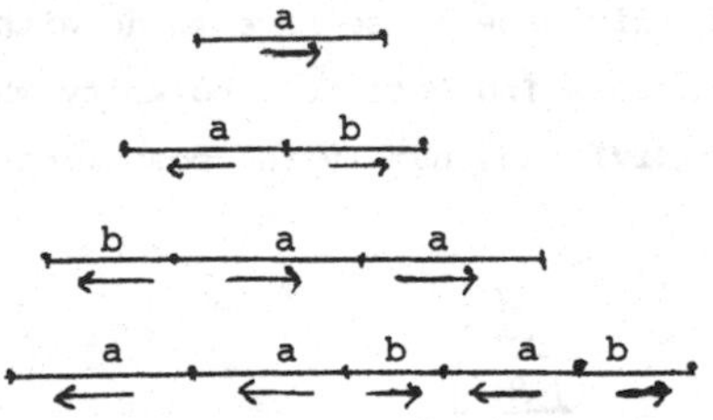

The following two edge production rules are sufficient:

$$a \rightarrow a^{-}\ b^{+}$$

$$b \rightarrow a^{+}$$

Clearly this kind of systems of productions could be defined on any set of directed and labeled graphs, but for biological reasons we prefer to consider only certain restricted types of graphs.

First of all we wish to extend this formalism to branching structures. The following example of a developmental sequence of branching filaments may be considered. Such sequence can be found in many algae and fungi.

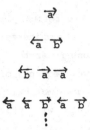

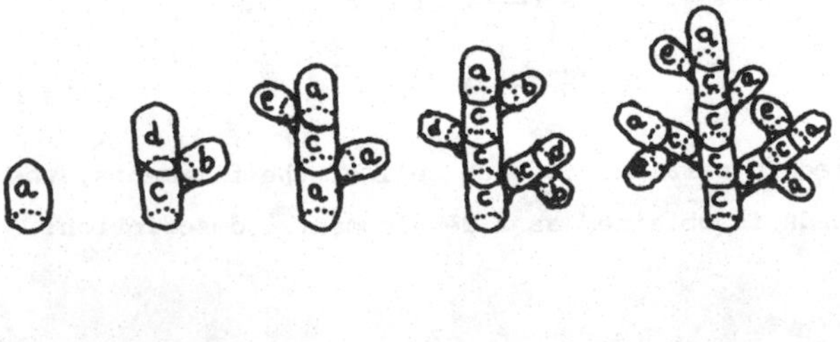

The symbols a, b, c, d, e indicate again cytological states, related to the timing of cell divisions, and polarity is present (but not shown) upward or outward along the branches in a natural orientation for a plant structure. Note that some of the division walls are transverse to the filament on which they occur, and some are in a lateral position, where a branch is attached. Also, there is branching to the right and to the left of the mother branch, the entire structure lying flat on the plane.

In a formal-language-theoretical notation we again combine the cytological and polarity symbols. We also use round and square parentheses to indicate the direction of left and right branching directions. If a symbol is not included in parantheses then the corresponding cell is assumed to lie in the direction of the original filament. We have the following rewriting rules:

$$\vec{a} \longrightarrow \vec{c}\,\overrightarrow{[b]}\,\vec{d}$$
$$\vec{b} \longrightarrow \vec{a}$$
$$\vec{c} \longrightarrow \vec{c}$$
$$\vec{d} \longrightarrow \vec{c}\,\overrightarrow{(e)}\,\vec{a}$$
$$\vec{e} \longrightarrow \vec{d}$$

Since all arrows point in the same direction, we omit them from the notation, and obtain the following developmental sequence:

$$a$$
$$c[b]d$$
$$c[a]c(e)a$$
$$c[c[b]d]c(d)c[b]d$$
$$c[c[a]c(e)a]c(c(e)a)c[a]c(e)a$$
$$\vdots$$

The same development can be described in the graph-theoretical notation by using edge labels with + or - signs in the production rules as before, and in addition introducing branching markers $\uparrow$, $\downarrow$ to indicate edge insertion to the left or right the original edge (seen in the direction of its polarity). In parentheses after the markers we give the states and orientation symbols of the branches to be inserted. The production rules are then written in the following manner:

$$a \longrightarrow c^{+} \downarrow (b^{+})\ d^{+}$$
$$b \longrightarrow a^{+}$$
$$c \longrightarrow c^{+}$$
$$d \longrightarrow c^{+} \uparrow (e^{+})\ a^{+}$$
$$e \longrightarrow d^{+}$$

The following sequence of tree structures is obtained:

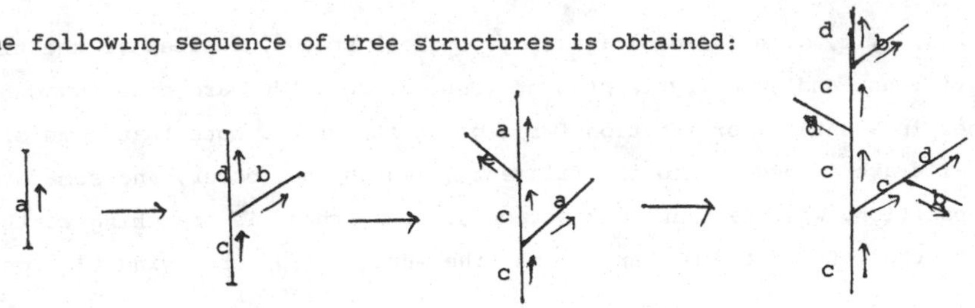

The distinction between the straight and lateral orientation of the edges is maintained. For this reason these tree structures are not the usual graph-theoretical trees in which all edges leaving a branching node are equivalent. In botanical trees there can be more than one lateral edge at each node, but there is at most one straight edge leaving each node. The markers used here distinguish only between the left and right pointing side branches. With more markers more orientations can be introduced if necessary.

The examples considered have to do with simple or branching filaments, which are essentially one-dimensional structures. If we wish to extend our theory to the development of 2-or 3-dimensional cellular structures, then only the graph-theoretical formalism appears to be feasible.

In the 2-dimensional case we have to consider sets of adjacent "walls" (faces) which share edges. Such a structure is called a "map". A map is a planar graph embedded in the plane with all vertices and edges lying on the boundaries of walls. The boundary of a wall consists of a circular sequence of edges. Edges are labelled and oriented. These edge labels and orientations are the main control factors in the generating systems to be considered.

Edge production rules are to be of the same form as before. Let us consider for instance the following set of rules for a map generating system

$$a \rightarrow \uparrow(a^-)\ b^+$$
$$b \rightarrow c^+ \uparrow(a^+)\ d^+$$
$$c \rightarrow e^+$$
$$d \rightarrow a^+$$
$$e \rightarrow f^+ \downarrow(a^+)$$
$$f \rightarrow c^+ \uparrow(a^+)\ g^+$$
$$g \rightarrow a^+ \downarrow(a^-)$$

Let the starting map be :

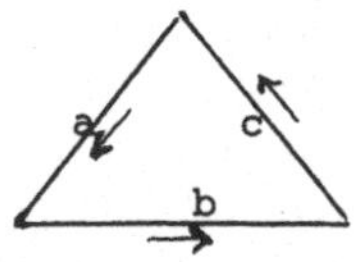

In a derivation step first the edges are to be rewritten according to the rules, and then a new edge is to be inserted if there are matching markers available inside a wall. Edge rewriting on the starting map yields an intermediate structure, and edge insertion results in the next map:

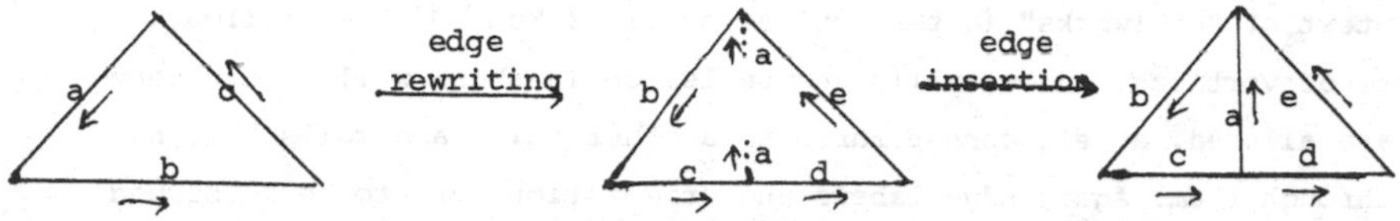

The following derivation steps result in a sequence of maps with triangular walls such that from a pair of sister walls one always divides in the first subsequent step and the other in the next step.

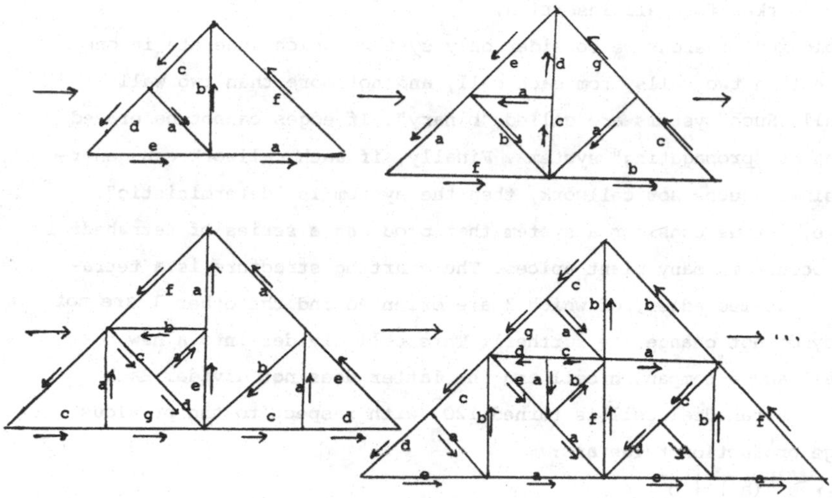

map sequence generated by above system.

It is easy to show that this derivation can go on infinitely with pairs of markers of matching labels or no markers produced on each wall. The markers outside the walls cannot be used. Unused markers are erased after the computation of the derivation step is completed (or, alternately, they can be saved for a certain number of steps). This is a deterministic derivation, each map has a single successor. If more than 2 compatible markers are produced on a wall, then the derivation becomes non-deterministic even if the set of production rules is not. Orientation specification is necessary for all labels with eventually non-palindromic derivations.

We see that there is no difference in the definition of production rules between 1- and 2-dimensional context-free systems, only the derivation definition is more complex in the latter case because edge insertion has to be defined with a search for matching markers.

Progressing to 3-dimensional cellular development, we consider them in the context of "cellworks" (a term coined by Liu & Fu [47]). A cellwork consists of vertices, edges, walls and cells. Cells share walls. Only convex cells are allowed, a cell cannot surround another cell, and cells have no holes through them. Again edge labels and orientations are to be construed as the sole control factors for the generation of new cellworks. In such a generating system not only the edges have to be rewritten and new edges have to be inserted, but it also has to be specified where new walls are inserted. The position of a new wall can be specified within the "shell" of the cell into which it has to be inserted. This shell is in fact a map, on which certain edges are marked for wall insertion.

For biological reasons we consider only systems which generate in one step not more than two cells from each cell, and not more than two walls from each wall. Such systems are called "binary". If edges cannot be erased then we speak of "propagating" systems. Finally, if each cellwork can generate only a single successor cellwork, then the system is "deterministic". As an example, let us consider a system that produces a series of tetrahedral cells as it occurs in many plant apices. The starting structure is a tetrahedron with 6 labeled edges, of which 3 are oriented and the other 3 are not (because they do not change any further). This cell divides into a new tetrahedral cell and a companion cell and the latter does not divide. Each division of a tetrahedral cell is turned 120° with respect to the previous one. The edge production rules are:

$$a \longrightarrow e \mid (a^-) \mid (b^-)\ c^-$$

$$b \longrightarrow e \mid (b^+) \mid (d)\ d$$

$$c \longrightarrow e \mid (a^+) \mid (d)\ d$$

$$d \longrightarrow d$$

$$e \longrightarrow e$$

We use vertical lines, instead of arrows, as markers because in 3 dimensions there are not only two but as many directions in which the new edges can be inserted as there are walls adjacent to the edge being rewritten. On which of these walls is the new edge to be inserted is specified by the wall production rules where the underlined edge symbols designate the newly inserted edge.

$$a^+\ c^-\ d \longrightarrow \underline{a^+}\ \ c^-\ d,\ \underline{a^-}\ e\ d\ e$$

$$b^-\ d\ c^+ \longrightarrow \underline{d}\ d\ d,\ \underline{d}\ e\ d\ e$$

$$b^+\ a^-\ d \longrightarrow \underline{b^-}\ d\ c^+,\ \underline{b^+}\ e\ d\ e$$

These 3 wall productions program the splitting of a wall into two new walls. Changes in wall configurations which do not involve the production of two new walls do not need to be specified since they follow directly from the edge rewriting. Each wall is described by a circular sequence of edge labels and orientation signs. This sequence is meant to be read in the clockwise direction on each wall as viewed from within each cell type. Above we give the edge sequences from the point of view of the tetrahedral cells.

It is the cell production rule which determines where the division wall is to be inserted. This rule is:

$$(a^+c^-d,\ b^-dc^+,\ b^+a^-d,\ ddd) \rightarrow$$
$$\rightarrow (a^+c^-d,\ b^-dc^+,\ \underline{b^+a^-d},\ ddd),\ (\underline{b^-da^+},\ dede,\ a^-ede,\ b^+ede,\ ddd)$$

Each cell (shown in parentheses) is described by its set of walls. The wall to be inserted is underlined in both daughter cells. Note that the circular sequences b^+a^-d and b^-da^+ designate the same wall, looked at from different daughter cells. A derivation step consists of three consecutive structures, they are generated first by edge rewriting, then by edge insertion, and finally by wall insertion.

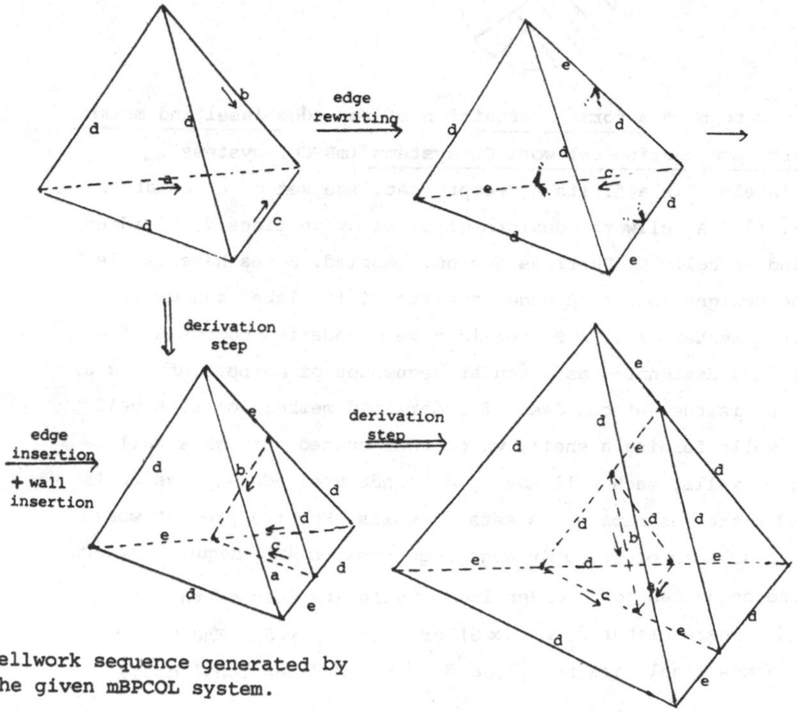

cellwork sequence generated by
the given mBPCOL system.

In the next derivation steps the tetrahedral cells divide again and again, and the companion cells do not but they are transformed to new configurations. For this process we need the following additional wall production rules, written from the point of view of the companion cells (they are mirror image descriptions of the walls found in the last 2 wall productions given above).

$$b^-da^+ \rightarrow \underline{b^+c^-d},\ \underline{b^-}\ ede$$
$$b^+c^-d \rightarrow \underline{ddd},\ \underline{d}\ ede$$

By these rules the cellwork of the next derivation step and of all further ones are produced. Some of the non-dividing cells, and their walls, change their edge configurations during these steps, these changes can be directly obtained by the edge rewriting rules.

The rules listed above: 5 edge productions, 5 wall productions and a single cell production, completely specify an infinite sequence of turning tetrahedral divisions by which 3 growing ranks of non-dividing cells are produced. The growth of this pattern proceeds with the tetrahedral apical cell being always at the bottom, such as one would see in a growing root. A two-dimensional version of such a growth pattern (producing 2 ranks of companion cells) is shown below.

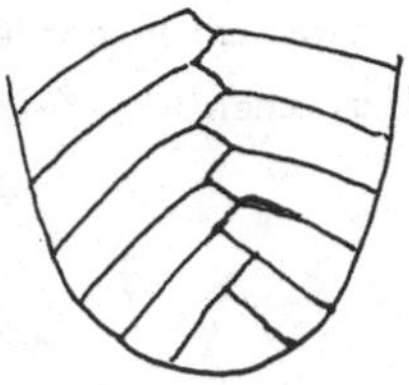

We proceed now to give <u>a formal definition of the edge-label and marker controlled, binary, propagating cellwork OL-systems</u> (mBPCOL-systems). The set of edge labels Σ is a finite non-empty set. The set of orientation signs S is $\{+, -, \underline{+}\}$. A cellwork consists of a set of vertices V, of edges E, of walls W, and of cells C. Vertices are not labeled. Edges have labels and polarity. The designation of an edge consists of its label and orientation sign, it is a member of $(\Sigma \times S)$. Walls have boundaries composed of edges, walls are thus designated as circular sequences of members of $(\Sigma \times S) \cup (\Sigma_u \times S)$ where Σ_u is the set composed of underlined members of Σ. A cell is surrounded by walls forming a shell, which when opened through a wall is a map consisting of walls, each wall having a boundary of edges. Thus cells can be designated either as maps or as sets of walls. For the present work we designate cells as sets of circular edge sequences, anyone sequence written as σ_i, some of these sequences to be underlined. Cells are sets of the form $\{\sigma_1, \sigma_2, \ldots, \sigma_n\}$, where either $\sigma_i \in (\Sigma \times S)$ or $\sigma_i \in (\Sigma_u \times S)$. The set M of markers in the 3-dimensional case is $\{|\}$, and in the 2-dimensional case $\{\downarrow, \uparrow\}$.

An mBPCOL-system consists of

(1) a set EP of edge productions,

(2) a set WP of wall productions,

(3) a set CP of cell productions, and

(4) a starting cellwork ω,

EP is a set of pairs of the form $a \to x$, where $a \in \Sigma$ and $x \in [(\Sigma \times S) \cup (M \times \Sigma \times S)]^*$

WP is a set of pairs of the form $w_1 \rightarrow (w_2, w_3)$ where w_1 is a circular sequence of members of $(\Sigma \times S)$, and w_2, w_3 are circular sequences of members of $(\Sigma \times S) \cup (\Sigma_u \times S)$. In each of the sequences w_2, w_3 there is exactly one member of $(\Sigma_u \times S)$, indicating the newly inserted edge.
CP is a set of pairs of the form $c_1 \rightarrow (c_2, c_3)$, where c_1 is a set consisting of walls which are defined as circular sequences of members of $(\Sigma \times S)$, and c_2, c_3 are sets consisting of walls which are circular sequences either of members of $(\Sigma \times S)$ or of members of $(\Sigma_u \times S)$.

In each of the sets c_2 and c_3 there is exactly one underlined sequence of edges, indicating the division wall.

A derivation step of an mBPCOL-system, producing cellwork X_2 from cellwork X_1, consists of 3 stages. First, all edges of X_1 are rewritten in a parallel way by the application of the rules in EP, thereby producing structure X_1'. Secondly, new edges are inserted on all the walls on which two matching markers are present and for which a rule is available in WP. In this way structure X_1'' is obtained. Thirdly, new walls are inserted in cells of which the shell contains a circular sequence of underlined edges and for which a rule is available in CP. Thereby the cellwork X_2 is generated.

A derivation consists of finitely many derivation steps. If the system is deterministic, i.e., in each step a single cellwork is generated from the previous one, then a derivation sequence (developmental sequence) is obtained beginning with the starting cells. Otherwise a derivation tree is obtained, and the set of all cellworks generated including the starting cellwork, forms a developmental language.

Clearly, the above definition of cellwork generating systems is suitable to serve as the basis for the definitions of the preceding graph-theoretically introduced 1- and 2-dimensional generating systems. The main difference in the notation between the 2-dimensional branching or map systems on the one hand, and the 3-dimensional systems on the other hand lies in the fact that in 2 dimensions each edge can have only two adjacent walls while in 3 dimensions more than two walls may be adjacent to an edge. Thus in the former case 2 markers are sufficient, while in the latter either many markers have to be adopted, or a single marker but with additional wall and cell productions. In our formal definition we chose the latter convention. In the truly 1-dimensional case (unbranched filaments) no markers are needed. Obviously, in the derivations of unbranched or branched filaments no edge insertions need to be carried out, and in the derivations of maps no wall insertions are needed.

These graph-theoretical definitions can easily be extended to systems with interactions among the edges (context-sensitive rewriting). Since each edge coincides with 2 vertices and has an orientation, one may speak of a left and right context to each edge. These contexts consist of the sets of labels and signs belonging to the edges which share the left- or right-hand vertex of a given edge. Thus the edge labeled a in the diagram has left-context α and right-context β.

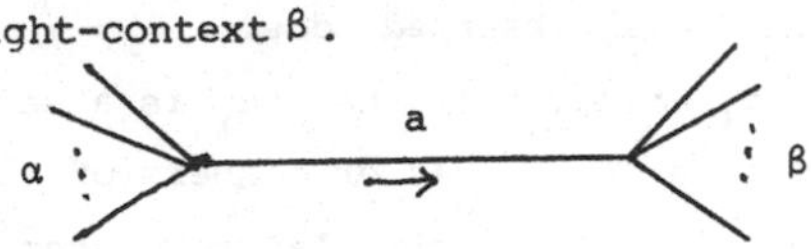

The edge productions are then of the form:

$(\alpha, a, \beta) \rightarrow x$

where $\alpha, \beta \subseteq (\Sigma \cup S)$, $a \in \Sigma$, and $x \in (\Sigma \cup S)^*$. This type of context-sensitive map systems has been considered in [57].

Similarly, our definitions could be extended to cover non-propagating systems. In other words, edge erasing would be allowed. Two variants of such systems come immediately to mind. In one, erasing of an edge would result in the disconnection of its two vertices. This may result in the structure falling apart, which has been considered by Ruohonen [67a] in the definition of JL-systems. The other possibility is to contract the disappearing edge in such a way that its two vertices come to coincide. This would result in the shrinkage of the structures, without their falling apart, which would be convenient for many biological applications (especially since a disconnected structure cannot be connected again under our basic assumptions that edges are generated only from edges and not from vertices and that new edges are generated only between markers within the same wall). The latter convention has also been considered in [58].

Finally, the requirement for binary cell and wall divisions could also be reconsidered, but there is no biological motivation for abandoning this requirement and it would introduce such complications that it is better to be maintained.

The generating systems presented here are in fact parallel graph grammars, i.e., they generate sequences or sets of edge-labeled and directed graphs by means of edge rewriting. But our definitions cover only four categories of graphs, namely linear graphs, trees (more precisely: "botanical trees", with a distinction between straight lateral attachment of branches), maps, and cellworks. In graphs which do not fall under one of these categories one could also carry out edge rewriting, and thereby generate new graphs, but one would not have any rules for the insertion of new edges or walls (since these insertion rules depend on the definitions of walls and cells, and graphs in general do not have such elements).

We should note that the biological interpretation of a labeled edge is different in the 1-, 2-, or 3-dimensional structures. In the 1-dimensional case (linear and tree graphs) the edge labels represent cell states. In the

2-dimensional case (maps) the edge labels stand actually for wall states. In 3-dimensions only represent edge labels states of the edges themselves. This change of representation has resulted in ambiguities in the terminology used in previous articles (for instance, edges were called "walls" and walls "cells" in [46]). Other types of map and cellwork systems lack the markers and use circular words as main control devices [13, 44a, 46].

Another kind of graph-theoretical definitions of L-systems was considered in [11, 12, 45, 55, 56] with both node- and edge-labeled rewriting (graph L-systems). They were based on node substitutions and many useful results are available for them, some of which being applicable to the constructs presented here (or their duals). The main difficulty with these systems is that they rewrite graphs from which the cellular structures cannot be recovered in an unambiguous way.

The formal-language-theoretical definitions of L-systems are presented next. These definitions are given for linear arrays of symbols (words). Their extension to branching arrays of symbols has also been considered [39].

An interactionless L-system (OL-system) is a triple $G = (\Sigma, P, \omega)$, where Σ is a finite nonempty set (of cell states), P is a mapping from Σ into Σ^*, and ω is an element of Σ^+. We write an element of P (a cell state production rule) as $a \rightarrow x$, where $a \in \Sigma$ and $x \in \Sigma^*$. We say that string x directly derives string y in the OL system G, and write $x \underset{G}{\Rightarrow} y$, if there is an integer $n \geq 1$ and there are symbols a_i and strings p_i, for $1 \geq i \geq n$, such that

$$x = a_1\, a_2 \ldots a_n$$

$$y = p_1\, p_2 \ldots p_n$$

and for every i, $a_i \rightarrow p_i$ is a production of G. Furthermore, we say that string x derives string y in G, and write $x \underset{G}{\overset{*}{\Rightarrow}} y$, if there are strings $q_0, q_1, \ldots q_n$, for some integer $n \geq 0$, such that

$$q_0 \underset{G}{\Rightarrow} q_1 \underset{G}{\Rightarrow} q_2 \underset{G}{\Rightarrow} \ldots \underset{G}{\Rightarrow} q_n$$

and $x = q_0$ and $y = q_n$.

The language generated by an OL-system $G = (\Sigma, P, \omega)$, denoted as $L(G)$, is $L(G) = \{x \mid \omega \underset{G}{\overset{*}{\Rightarrow}} x\}$. The sequence of strings generated by a deterministic OL-system $G = (\Sigma, P, \omega)$, denoted as $E(G)$, is $E(G) = x_0, x_1, x_2, \ldots$ where $x_0 = \omega$ and $x_i \underset{G}{\Rightarrow} x_{i+1}$ for every $i \geq 0$. Such a sequence may be finite, if the last string in the sequence is the empty string, otherwise it is infinite.

The definition of interactive L-systems (IL-systems) takes account of certain numbers of left and right neighbour cell states and of environmental symbols at both ends of the strings. A system is a (k,ℓ) L-system if k left neighbours (or environmental symbols) and ℓ right neighbours (or environmental symbols) are to be taken into account in determining the substitution for a given cell, in addition to the state of the cell itself. We assume, in the simplest case, that there is a single environmental symbol g in sufficient copies to the left and right of each string to make derivation possible. In cases where environmental variation is desired, certain sequences of different environmental symbols may be specified.

A (k,ℓ) L-system is a four-tuple $G = (\Sigma, P, g, \omega)$, where Σ is a finite nonempty set of symbols, P is a mapping from $(\Sigma \cup \{g\})^k x \Sigma x (\Sigma \cup \{g\})^\ell$ into Σ^*, g is a symbol not in Σ, and $\omega \in \Sigma^+$. The elements of P (productions) are written in the form $(w_1, a, w_2) \rightarrow w_3$, where $a \in \Sigma$, $w_1 \in (\Sigma \cup \{g\})^k$, $w_2 \in (\Sigma \cup \{g\})^\ell$ and $w_3 \in \Sigma^*$. The strings w_1 and w_2 must also satisfy the following conditions:

(i) if $w_1 = w_1' \, g \, w_1''$ for some w_1' and $w_1'' \in (\Sigma \cup \{g\})^*$, then $w_1' \in \{g\}^*$;

(ii) if $w_2 = w_2' \, g \, w_2''$ for some w_2' and $w_2'' \in (\Sigma \cup \{g\})^*$, then $w_2'' \in \{g\}^*$.

Furthermore, a completeness condition is required, namely that for every triple (w_1, a, w_2) from $(\Sigma \cup \{g\})^k \times \Sigma \times (\Sigma \cup \{g\})^\ell$, such that w_1 and w_2 satisfy conditions (i) and (ii), there exists a string $w_3 \in \Sigma^*$ such that $(w_1, a, w_2) \rightarrow w_3$ is an element of P.

In the derivation of a string y from a string x under a (k, ℓ) L-system we thus consider $(k + \ell + 1)$-tuples of cells for the computation of a new string to be substituted for each cell in x, and then concatenate these strings in the correct order to form string y. The definition for this procedure is analogous to that for OL-systems. The languages and sequences of interactive L-systems (systems for any k and ℓ larger than or equal to 0) can also be defined analogously to those for OL-systems.

Characterization

We would like to associate algebraic or analytical properties with various classes of L-systems, such as the OL, DOL, IL, DIL classes of systems. The most useful results would be those which require the existence of certain (finite) sets of structures in the sequence or language generated by a certain class of systems. On the basis of such testable properties one could rule out the possibility that a member of a given class of systems can generate certain naturally occurring patterns. Such a conclusion would help the search for the underlying biological mechanism for an observed developmental process. For instance, if OL-systems are ruled out as generators of certain developmental patterns, then either cell interactions (IL-systems) or environmental changes (table L-systems) would have to be considered.

The mathematical literature on L-systems that has accumulated over the past 18 years contains many results that can be used for characterization. We can only list a few of these results, and without proofs, but with references to the original publications.

Theorem (Rozenberg & Doucet [66]). Let $G = (\Sigma\ , P, \omega)$ be an OL-system. Then there exists a positive integer C_G such that every string x in L(G) has a derivation sequence in G, $x_0, x_1, x_2, \ldots x_n$, such that $x_0 = \omega$ and $x_n = x$, and for every i, $0 \le i \le n$, $\ell(x_i) \le C_G \quad (\ell(x) + 1)$. Here '$\ell(x)$' stands for the number of symbols in string x.

Theorem (Herman & Walker [24]). The class of adult languages of OL-systems (AOL-languages) is the same as the class of context-free languages. The adult (or stable) language of an OL-system G is defined as the set of strings generated by G each of which derives only itself under the productions of G.

There is a well-known partial characterization of the class of context--free languages, namely 'the pumping lemma' of Bar-Hillel [28]. By the above theorem, the classes of context-free and AOL-languages are identical, thus if a language L is an AOL-language it must satisfy the pumping property specified by the lemma. This result is mostly used in the form of its negation, i.e., if a set of strings (corresponding to adult structures of an organism) does not have this property then this set cannot be adult language of a string OL-system (these structures could not arise without interactions).

The relationship between classes of L-languages and classes of Chomsky-languages has been investigated in some detail (see Herman & Rozenberg [22]), as shown below.

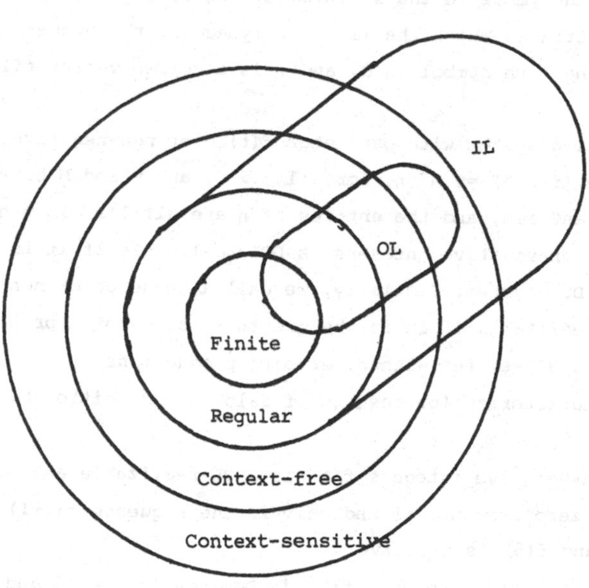

Intersections of OL and IL languages with Chomsky languages.

While the classes of DOL- and OL-languages are properly included in the set of context-sensitive languages, the class of IL-languages is not included. The classes of DOL- and OL-languages have non-empty intersections with the classes of regular, context-free and context-sensitive languages, and the class of IL-languages includes that of regular languages. These inclusion and exclusion properties, together with well-known results on Chomsky categories, help also to distinguish between languages or sequences which can be generated with or wihout cellular interactions.

Strong characterization results are available for the growth functions of DOL-systems. The growth function f(t) of a deterministic string L-system G is the number of cells $\ell(x_t)$ in the t-th string x_t in E(G).

In linear system theory, a system with observable parameter f(t) ranging over non-negative integers is called N-realizable if there is a π, M, η such that $f(t) = \pi M^t \eta$ for all $t \geq 0$, where π is a row vector, η is a column vector and M is a square matrix, all of the same dimension and all with non--negative integer entries. Similarly, a system is called Z-realizable if there exists such an expression with all integer entries.

The following observation of Paz and Salomaa [61] shows the connection of these terms to growth functions of DOL-systems. The growth function f(t) of a DOL-system G with k symbols can be written in the form $f_G(t) = \pi M^t \eta$ where π is a k-dimensional row vector whose i-th entry equals the number of occurrences of the i-th symbol in the starting string of G, M is a (k x k) dimensional square matrix in which the (i,j) entry equals the number of j-th symbols produced by the i-th symbol in G, and η is a column vector filled with 1's.

We therefore call a system with parameter f(t) over non-negative integers DOL-realizable if $f(t) = \pi M^t \eta$, for all $t \geq 0$, and π and M have all non-negative integer entries, and the entries of η are all 1's. In other words, a sequence of non-negative integers is DOL-realizable if it is the growth function of a DOL-system. Similarly, we call a sequence of non-negative integers PDOL-realizable if it is the growth function of a propagating DOL-system, i.e., of a DOL-system without erasing productions.

The following characterization results of Salomaa and Soittola [69] are then available.

(1) A sequence of non-negative integers f(t) is PDOL-realizable and not identical to the zero sequence if and only if the sequence f(t+1) - f(t) is N-realizable and f(0) is positive.

(2) For any integer $k \geq 0$, the sequence f(t) is DOL-realizable if and only if the sequence f(t+k) is DOL-realizable.

(3) If f(t) is a DOL-realizable sequence not becoming ultimately zero, then there is a constant c such that for all $t > 0$, $\frac{f(t+1)}{f(t)} \le c$.

(4) Every Z-realizable sequence of integers can be expressed in the form $f(t) = f_1(t) - f_2(t)$, where $f_1(t)$ and $f_2(t)$ are DOL-realizable sequences.

These and other theorems make it possible to decide whether an observed growth function of an organism is DOL-, resp. PDOL-realizable. Other theorems enable us to obtain explicit, polynomial and/or exponential, functions for given DOL-systems. Growth functions can also be found for each type of cell separately (the so-called Parikh-functions of L-systems) which can be used in ecological or crop growth studies.

Growth functions can also be obtained for the graph-theoretical and multidimensional L-systems. In the 3-dimensional case, we can ask for growth functions of cells, walls or edges. In the various edge-label systems the most interesting questions concern the edge growth functions. Such growth functions are obviously DOL-realizable functions in the case of interactionless one-dimensional systems (simple and branching filaments). For map OL--systems the edge growth functions are more complex because of the edge insertion operations. It has been shown [13], however, that the edge and wall growth functions of binary propagating map DOL-systems are also DOL-realizable.

Inference

The problem of finding L-systems which generate an observed sequence of structures is called their "syntactic inference" problem. In fact it could also be called their "realization" problem. We are faced here with a more difficult type of realization then in the previous section where the problem was to realize the growth function of a developmental process, i.e., the sequence of its numbers of cells or edges. Now we are asking for the realization of the sequence of the structures themselves.

The following cases have been considered [13c, 20, 22, 23, 70] for the inference problem of string-generating OL-systems: (a) all intervals between observations equal 1, (b) all intervals between observations are equal but of unknown length, (c) the intervals are of arbitrary lengths but the observations are in the proper order. Both deterministic (D) and non-deterministic, propagating (P) and non-propagating systems ere considered, as well as the presence and absence of cell interactions (2, 1, and 0 sided interactions). The inference problem was shown to be decidable for the cases Dax, Dbx (x = 0, 1, 2) and for Dc2, while the decidability has not been proven for the cases Dc0 and Dc1, and not even for PDc1.

Recently the DOL inference problem has been considered for branching filaments [33]. Plant branching structures have usually an unlimited development, i.e., the termination of their development is caused by external factors, not by internal programming. The branch apices have a large degree of autonomy, in other words their development often does not depend on signals received from other parts of the plant. Furthermore, the fate of each branch apex can be easily followed, and its daughter branches identified. Under these conditions it is possible to construct an algorithm to find the set of DOL-systems (with branching symbols) which generate a given (finite) sequence of branching structures.

This algorithm first assigns different symbols to each apex and then finds the lineage trees (trees of descendants) for the labeled apices. On these lineage trees isomorphic subtrees are then identified and the apices are relabeled in such a way that corresponding apices receive the same label. Among the trees obtained other isomorphisms may be found, and the corresponding portions again relabeled. The algorithm stops when no further isomorphism can be found. At that point the remaining labels are considered to be the state symbols of a DOL-system, and the descent relations among them the productions of that system. The algorithm is non-deterministic, since by another choice of isomorphisms among the lineages another DOL-system may be obtained. Among all such systems obtained we can ask for the ones with minimum number of symbols or with productions of a certain form. Also, additional criteria may be applied by which the most desirable (from a biological point of view) system is chosen. We can also state criteria which make systems unacceptable, for instance if they need too many symbols in proportion to the size of structures. If no acceptable DOL-systems are provided by the algorithm then this should be taken as an indication that other types of generating systems should be considered, such as stochastic OL-systems, table OL-systems, or IL-systems. The inference problem for stochastic OL-system has been investigated by Nishida [60] with reference to the development of Japanese cypress shoots. In stochastic OL-systems several productions may be present for the same symbol [15a,32] and probability distribution has to be found for each set of such productions. Each probability distribution involves one or more parameters the values of which must be estimated from observations. For one or a few parameters this may be possible , but not for as many as in the case of the cypresses. A stochastic OL-system with a single probabilistic parameter was applied to cell division rates in roots [21a].

Stochastic OL-systems with tables were studied by Jürgensen [32] and Jürgensen, Matthews & Wood [34], and their inference problems by Schmidt [70]. No general algorithms have been constructed yet for the inference problem of stochastic L-systems. Similarly, the inference problem of IL-systems appears to be quite difficult, except in the cases where only one signal is involved, and only a few parameters need to be estimated.

Complexity

Since L-systems have a biological interpretation, differences between their complexities have also direct biological meaning. If systems can be identified with a minimum measure of computational complexity to generate certain developmental patterns then we can speak in fact of minimalization results concerning the necessary control factors. Organisms do not in general minimalize their energy expenditures, or their information storage capacities, but they might have acquired minimal control system constructions by selection and evolution. Each additional cellular state has to arise and be maintained by involved biochemical and physiological mechanisms, so it is to the advantage of the organism to keep the number of discrete steady states as low as possible. Similarly, each time a signal has to be produced in a certain cell, transmitted over a number of other cells, and finally received and recognized by still other cells, many cell components have to be synthetized and transported. Thus it is reasonable to assume that the number of states and signals has been selected so that duplications are avoided.

Within formal language theory two main measures of complexity can be distinguished. First, there is the decidability of certain questions, such as membership, emptiness, equivalence, with respect to given classes of generating systems. Clearly, undecidability of certain questions in a given class indicates a higher complexity of that class than those in which the question is decidable. Once the decidability of a question has been proven, the second measure has to do with the computational complexity of the decision procedure, mostly expressed in terms of Turing machine time or space complexity values. There are other types of complexity comparisons possible. For instance, there is complexity in terms of number of subwords, or number of states, or number of state transitions, or number of levels in state graphs. The latter measures are very useful for comparisons among closely related systems.

We mention here first of all some of the decidability results for L--systems.

Growth function and Parikh equivalence is decidable for DOL sequences (Paz & Salomaa [61]).

The membership, finiteness, emptiness and equivalence problems are decidable for DOL sequences and languages (theorems by Rozenberg & Doucet [66], Culik & Fris [9]). The equivalence problems are concerned with the questions whether for any two DOL-systems G_1 and G_2 it is the case that $E(G_1) = E(G_2)$ and $L(G_1) = L(G_2)$, and were previously well-known open problems.

The equivalence problem is undecidable for the languages of OL-systems, even in the case of propagating systems (Blattner [5]).

The recently proven Ehrenfeucht conjecture (Albert & Lawrence [1], Semenov & Guba [71]) implies that the sequence equivalence question for HDOL and DTOL systems is decidable, which were open problems for some time. The former consist of homomorphisms of DOL-systems thus also of codings of DOL-systems (also called "CDOL-systems"). The latter are deterministic table OL-systems. While the sequence equivalence problem is decidable for these systems, the language equivalence problem is undecidable even for propagating DTOL-systems.

The sequence equivalence problem is undecidable for propagating D1L--systems (Vitányi [79]), while their membership problem is decidable.

There arise thus clearcut differences in decidabilities between the main classes: DOL, OL, DTOL, HDOL, TOL, DIL and IL systems with respect to the sequences and languages generated by them.

In those cases where the membership problem is decidable (all of the above classes except the IL), further questions can be posed about computational complexity. The upper bounds of Turing machine complexity are as follows (Jones & Skyum [30,31]):

	det. time compl.	det. tape complexity
PDOL	n (?)	-
DOL	n^2	$\log n$
OL	$n^{3.81}$	$\log^2 n$
DTOL	n^5 (?)	$\log^2 n$
TOL	NP-complete	n

Some results on subword complexity are as follows (Ehrenfeucht & Rozenberg [14,15]):

(1) For every DTOL language K over an alphabet with at least two symbols, the ratio of the number of different subwords of length k in words of K to the number of all possible words of length k over the same alphabet tends to 0 as k increases.

(2) For every DOL language K there is a constant c such that the number of subwords of K of length k is less than or equal to ck^2. This bound is the best possible one. For locally catenative DOL languages the bound is ck. For everywhere growing DOL languages the bound is $ck \log_2 k$. The latter two subclasses of DOL-systems are defined as follows.

A DOL-system G is locally catenative if the sequence $E(G) = x_1, x_2, \ldots$ satisfies the k-tuple $(i_1, i_2, \ldots, i_k)$ of positive integers with cut p, where p is an integer larger than the members of the k-tuple, if for all $n \geq p$:

$$x_n = x_{n-i_1} x_{n-i_2} \ldots x_{n-i_k}.$$

The locally catenative property of a DOL-system gives valuable insight into its recursiveness and is often directly observable on biological material. The observation of such recursive development is thus an indication that the sequence is realizable by a DOL-system. On the other hand, the decidability of locally catenativenees of an arbitrary DOL-system is a long-standing open problem. [37, 67, 68] .

A DOL-system is everywhere growing if the right-hand sides of all its productions contain more than one symbol. This type of system is not encountered too often because it lacks delay loops. We see that within the class of DOL-systems the introduction of the above two restrictions affects drastically the bounds of the number of subwords which occur in words of a given length and thus the bounds are complexity measures for these subclasses. For DTOL-systems no such bound is known, only that the number of subwords increases at a negligible rate in comparison to that of all possible subwords.

Finally, complexity classes have been proposed based on the state transition graphs of DOL-systems (Vitányi [79], Kelemenová [36]). Such a graph exhibits the symbol-to-symbol transitions in a set of productions, and on this basis 4 kinds of symbols can be distinguished: mortal, recursive, monorecursive, and expanding. The occurrence of some of these kinds of symbols in a DOL-system is associated with the nature of its growth function, which may be exponential, polynomial, limited or terminating. Since the growth function of a developmental process is mostly observable, one can use the association between growth functions and DOL-system properties to arrive at conclusions about the underlying complexity of the process.

In summary, many results are available about complexity differences between various classes of developmental generating systems. Undoubtedly many more results could be obtained, especially with respect to multi-dimensional development. The complexity measures for L-systems are basically different from those based on information and entropy, or from Kolmogorov[38] complexity. The difference lies in the fact that here we are dealing with control factors for derivations taking place in time and space, i.e., with growing distributedsystems, while the Shannon information and Kolmogorov complexity concepts concern only constant-size structures. The application of information or entropy measures to processes of living organisms has never been succesful for the additional reason that these measures are defined for information transmission (communication) from source to receiver over a canal and in organisms these components are not identifiable. For instance, the information content of the entire DNA complement of a living cell is immensely large and there is no way of finding out how and what part of it is actually used during the life time of the cell. This is why it is more likely to find useful comparisons between complexities of different organisms by considering their basic functional units, the cells, and the changes occurring in these units, such as cell divisions, cell death, changes in steady states, and changes leading to differentiation. These considerations are clearly related to those of computational complexity, pointing to a deep connection between computation and development.

Applications

We include here a short review of the biological applications of L--systems and related modular models. Most of this work consists of computer simulations of the development of certain plants and plant organs, based on various physiological mechanisms for growth and differentiation. The principles of these simulation models are seldom attributed directly to the mathematical results discussed above but many of them are tacitly used in their construction. For instance, in the course of the construction of each modular model it has to be decided at an early state whether there are going to be interactions among the modules or not. This choice clearly influences the structure of the model, and the complexity of the output that one expects. Similarly, the topology of the growing structure has to be established from the start, and the kinds and directions of the interactions among the modules. For instance, the maximum number of neighbours that each module may have is always an important parameter of the model. It is much easier to construct a model by considering the topology separately from the other geometric aspects (lengths, angles) of the components than to try to set them up together, which is what most biologists tend to do. Inference and characterization results are also built in intuitively in various aspects of the models.

One developmental problem which was attacked early by means of L-systems was the heterocyst spacing problem in blue-green bacteria. We already referred to these organisms at the beginning of the section on definitions, showing a DOL-system with cells in two developmental stages (a and b) and two polarity states. This type of development is well established in various species, for instance in Anabaena cylindrica. Superimposed on this pattern of vegetative cells in the same species is the production of specialized cells, the heterocysts, at regular intervals along the filament. Only vegetative cells in the b state can turn into heterocysts. The question is how the regular spacing of heterocysts arises: in this species there are on the average 10 vegetative cells between 2 heterocysts, while the filament is expanding by cell divisions of vegetative cells, as shown in the figure below (from [54]).

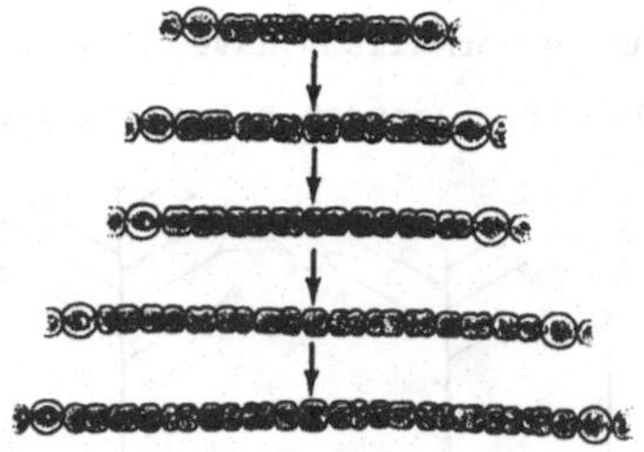

It is known that certain nitrogen-rich compounds are only produced in the heterocysts, so presumately the transport of these compounds regulates the appearance of heterocysts: where their concentration falls below a threshold value a vegetative cell (in state b) becomes induced: 2L-systems have been constructed for this process by Baker & Herman [3], and recently the mathematical properties of continuous vs. discrete models for this kind of development were investigated by de Koster & Lindenmayer [13b].

Branching plant structures are the most investigated developmental patterns so far. The stochastic model for vegetative shoots of the Japanese cypress (Chamaecyparis obtusa) by Nishida [60] has already been mentioned.

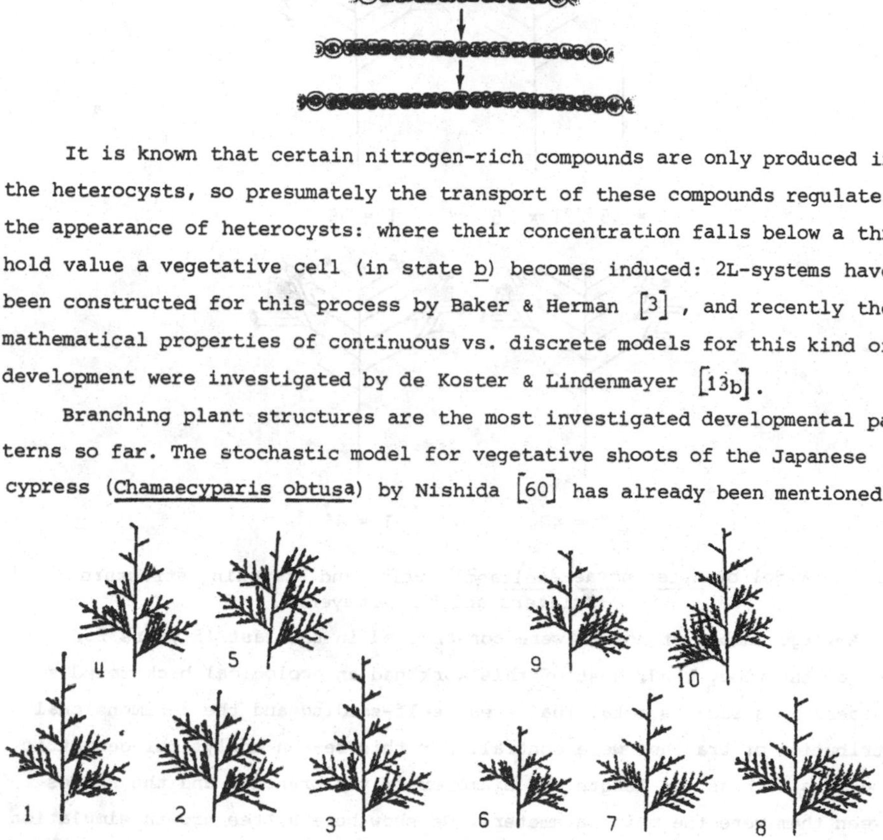

simulated shoots observed shoots
of the Japanese cypress

Several deterministic models with interactions have been produced for the flowering development of various Compositae members. We show here an early simulation of Aster novae-angliae with the timing and spacing of flowering heads as the most important aspect of the model (Frijters & Lindenmayer [18]). While the lengths of the stem segments are generated by the model (as state variables of the corresponding modules) the angles at which the branches are inserted are chosen in this case arbitrarily.

The main control factors are signals traveling upwards along the stems (essentially DIL-systems) and determining the time at which an apex is transformed from vegetative to flowering conditions. Other factors are the rates at which branch apices of various orders are producing side branches, and the rates at which the segments (internodes) grow (DOL-rules). Again, both discrete and continuous formalisms have been elaborated for flowering structures (Frijters [17 , 18], Janssen & Lindenmayer [29]).

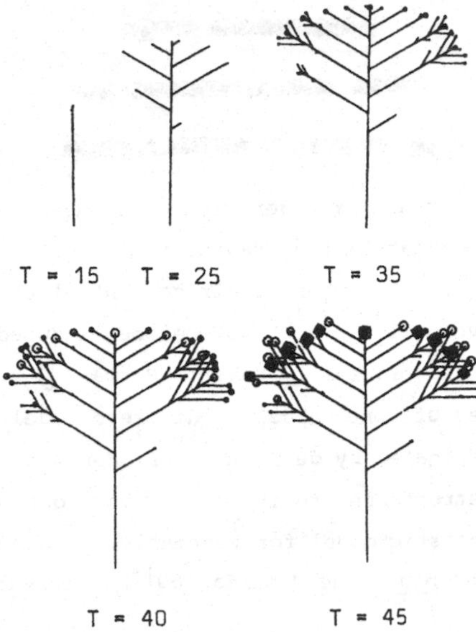

Model of <u>Aster novae-angliae</u> flowering and branching structure
(Frijters and Lindenmayer)

A large number of models were constructed in the last 15 years for trees of the woody kind. Most of this work had an ecological background so considerations such as total leaf area, self-shading and the 3-dimensional distribution of branches were contral. For this reason analytical-geometric properties such as the length and diameter of the branches and the angles between them were the main parameters. We show here a tree growth simulation by P. de Reffye & F. Hallé (personal communication, based on the book [21]) <u>Araucaria hunsteinii</u> where the production and shedding of branches and needles takes place according to a DOL-system, but the shapes of the branches are obtained by computing segment-by-segment the weight of the branch and the bending based on an elasticity coefficient. This coefficient is gradually changed from the bottom up, so that the top branches show less bending than the lower ones.

Other tree models were published by Honda [26], Fisher & Honda [16] , Honda, Tomlinson & Fisher [27], Borchert & Honda [6], among others. The mathematics of branching structures in general is the subject of a book by Macdonald [52].

Numerical relationships among components of branched organisms has been called "plant demography" and studied extensively by Harper, Bell and others [80]. Their expressions are related to the growth functions of L-systems with branching, primarily to the growth matrices of DOL-systems.

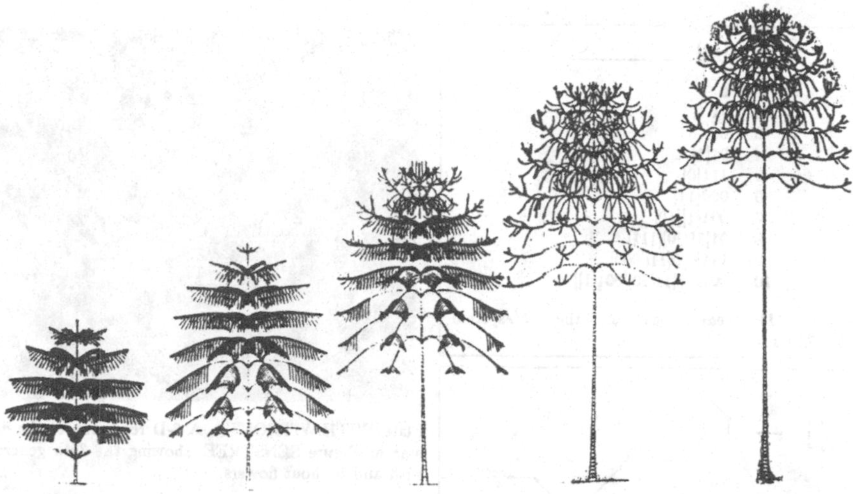

Araucaria hunsteinii developmental sequence (de Reffye & Hallé)

Recently computer graphics has evolved to the point that large trees, and even forests can be generated and exhibited on the screen. Such animated tree growth and forest graphics have been produced by Aono & Kunii [2] in Tokyo and by Smith [76] in San Francisco. We show here a few examples of their work.

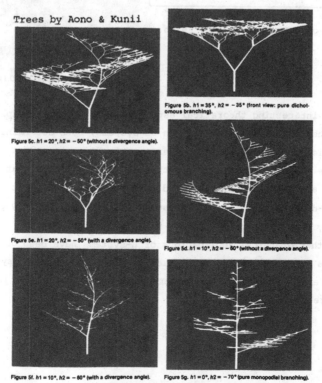

Trees by Aono & Kunii

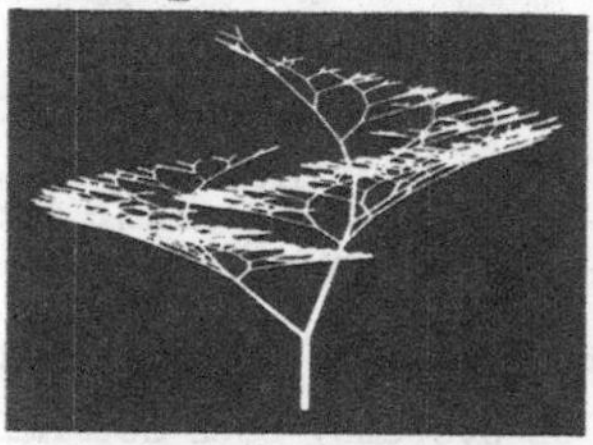

Figure 5c. $h1 = 20^\circ$, $h2 = -50^\circ$ (without a divergence angle).

Figure 5e. $h1 = 20^\circ$, $h2 = -50^\circ$ (with a divergence angle).

Figure 5f. $h1 = 10^\circ$, $h2 = -60^\circ$ (with a divergence angle).

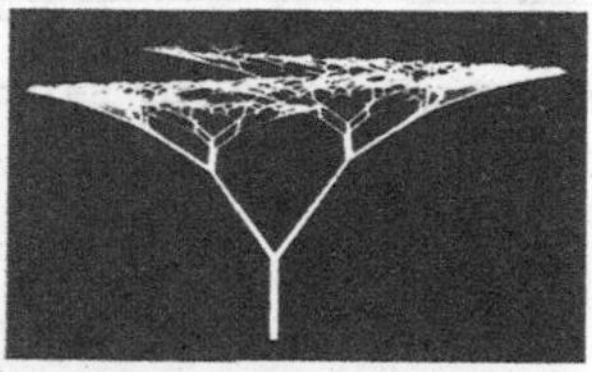

Figure 5b. $h1 = 35^\circ$, $h2 = -35^\circ$ (front view: pure dichotomous branching).

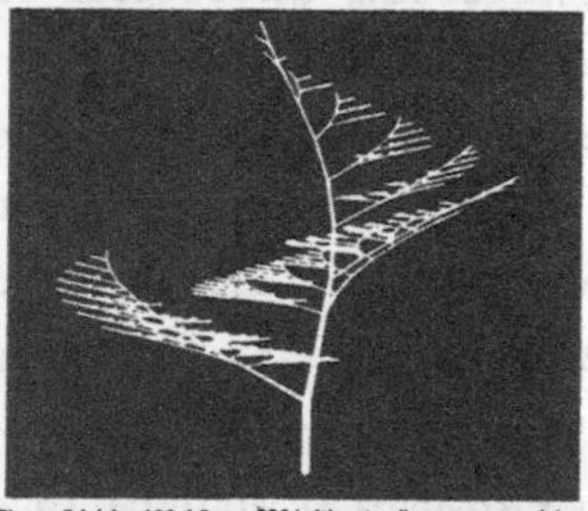

Figure 5d. $h1 = 10^\circ$, $h2 = -60^\circ$ (without a divergence angle).

Figure 5g. $h1 = 0^\circ$, $h2 = -70^\circ$ (pure monopodial branching).

n	L(n)
0	1
1	0
2	11
3	00
4	01[1]
5	111[0]
6	000[11]
7	001[1][10]
8	01[1]1[0][111]
9	111[0]0[11][000]
10	001[11]11[10][001[1]]

Table 1. 11 generations of the *2L*-system 0.1[1].1.1.0.11.1.0.

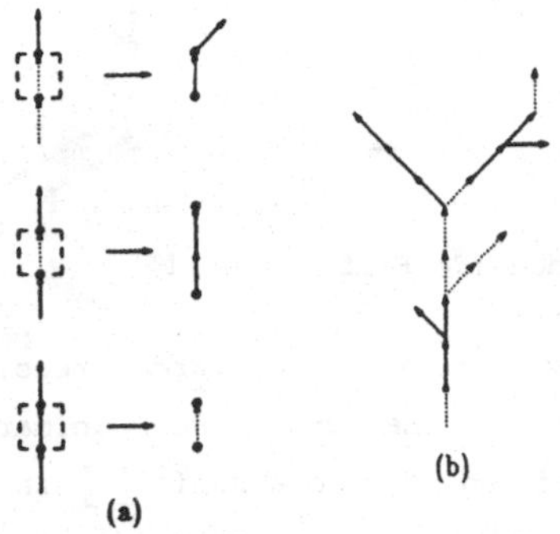

Figure SENSTREE. (a) Production rules. (b) Generation $n = 11$.

Computer graphics by Alvy Ray Smith.

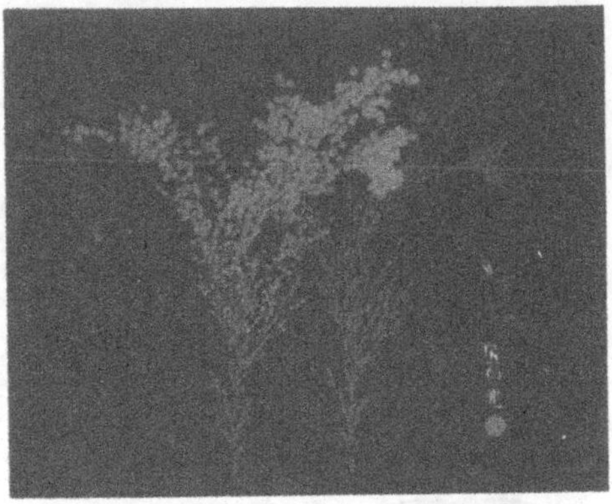

Plate WITH.WITHOUT. A 2-D rendering of the grammar in Figure SENSTREE, showing the 35th generation with and without flowers.

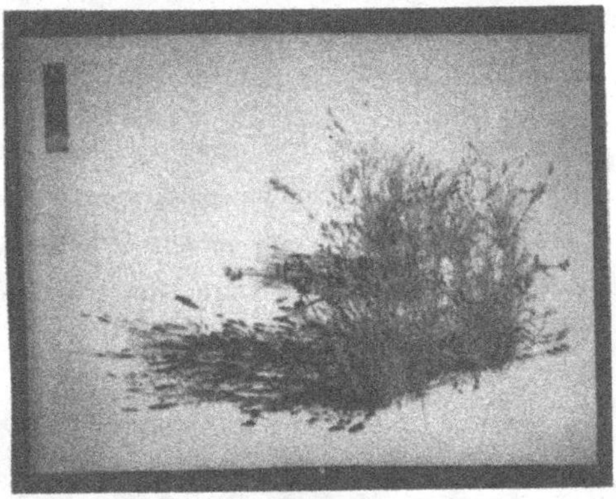

Plate WHITE.SANDS. Several 3-D renderings of the context-sensitive grammar 0.0.0.11.1.1[1].1.0 mixed with particle system grasses.

The interesting theoretical aspect of this creative graphics is that one of them is based essentially on OL-systems, both deterministic and stochastic, while the other on deterministic 2L-systems. Smith concludes about the "natural appearance" of the resulting pictures that the 2L--designs are more unpredictable and therefore more natural than the stochastic OL-designs. This is, of course, not surprising in view of the undecidability properties of the former which we have presented.

Further graphical applications of L-systems have been obtained by Szilard & Quinton [77] and Prusinkiewicz [62]. They use DOL-systems to draw line patterns under the turtle interpretation. Plant designs by the latter author are shown below.

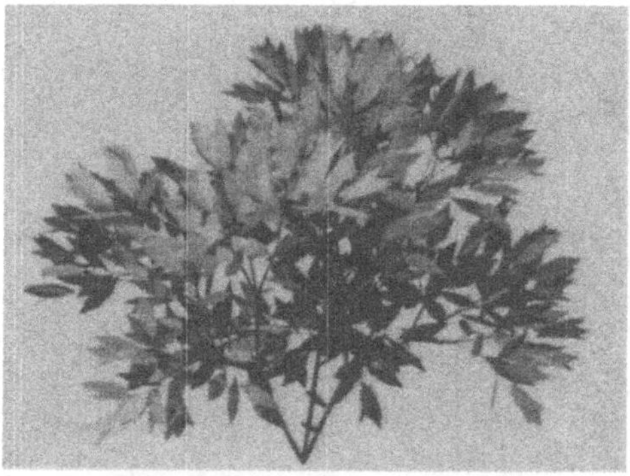

Fig. 3. The bush generated by L-system (4.2).

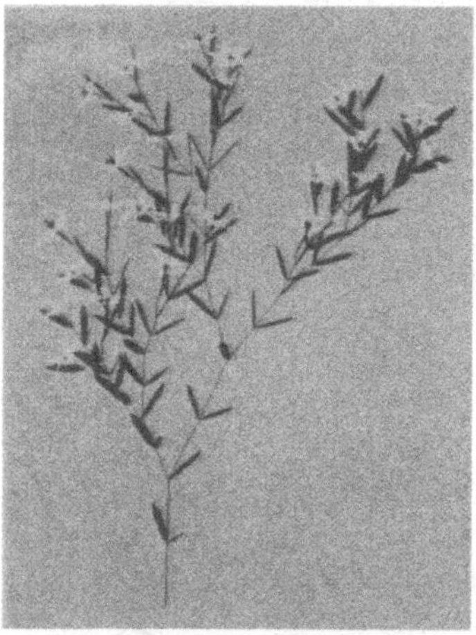

Fig. 4. The plant generated by L-system (4.4).

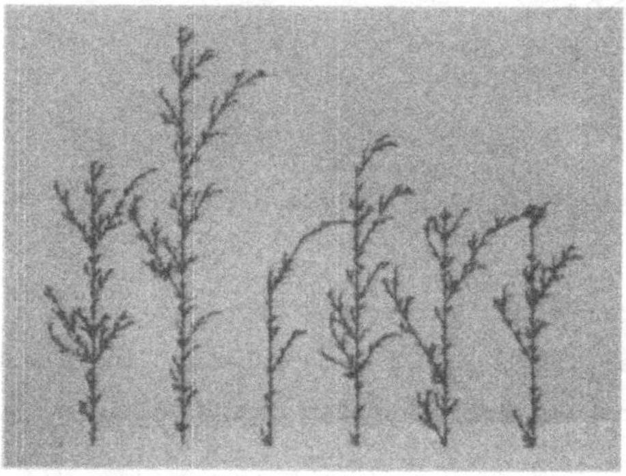

Fig. 5. Sample objects generated by the stochastic L-system (5.2).

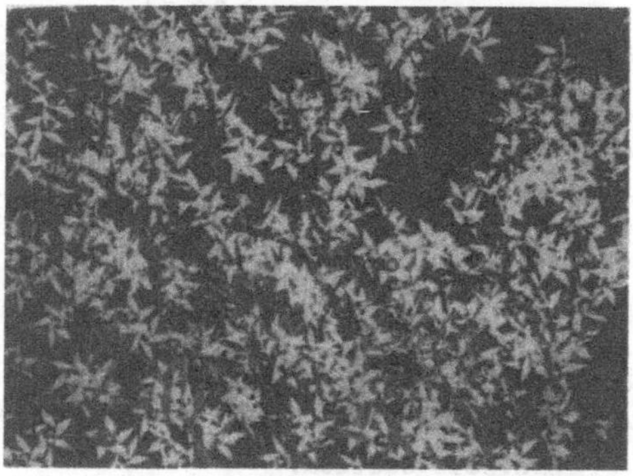

Fig. 6. The flower field.

Computer graphics by Prusinkiewicz

Finally, 2-dimensional generating algorithms have been applied to cell division patterns in leaf epidermis (Lück, Lindenmayer & Lück [49]) and to imaginal disc patterns in insects (Ransom [63], Matela & Ransom [51]). We show here an example of a moss leaf surface growth sequence generated by a map OL-system and drawn according to an algorithm with simple numerical rules determining the shapes and sizes of walls (from [13a]).

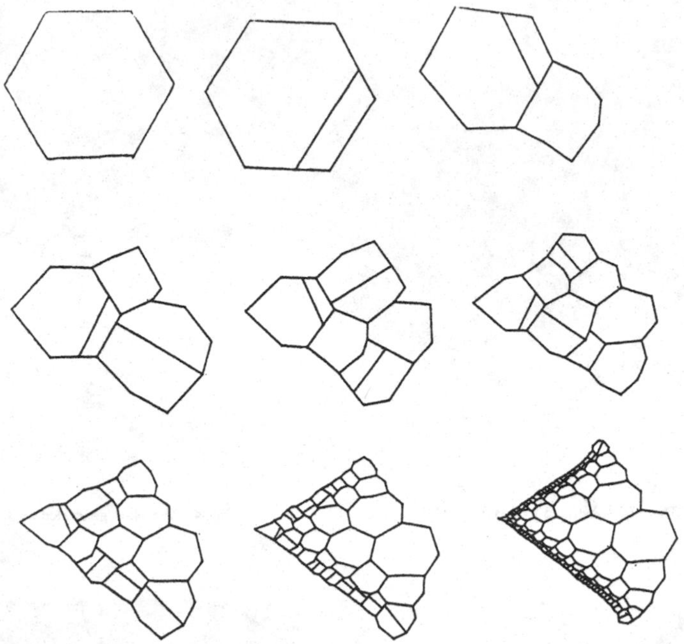

Moss leaf (Phascum cuspidatum) simulation by de Does & Lindenmayer.

The only 3-dimensional developmental model so far has been the one of the root apex of Azolla pinnata, a water fern [44] . The tetrahedral apical cell of such a root divides according to the mBPCOL-system presented in a previous section.

Multidimensional generating systems, with edge label control or other control factors, have many potential applications, also in architectural and landscape design, and represent a still largely unexplored territory.

References

1. M.H. Albert & J. Lawrence, A proof of Ehrenfeucht's conjecture. Theor. Comp. Sci., 41: 121-123, 1985.
2. M. Aono & T.L. Kunii, Botanical tree image generation. IEEE Computer Graphics & Appls., May 1984, pp. 10-34, 1984.
3. R. Baker & G.T. Herman, Simulation of organisms using a developmental model. Parts I & II. Int. J. Bio-Med. Computing, 3: 203-215, 251-267, 1972.

4. A.D. Bell, D. Roberts & A. Smith, Branching patterns: the simulation of plant architecture. J. Theor. Biol., 81: 351-375, 1979.
5. M. Blattner, The unsolvability of the equality problem for the sentential forms of context-free grammars. J. Comp. & Syst. Sci., 7: 463-468, 1973.
6. R. Borchert & H. Honda, Control of development in the bifurcating branch system of Tabebula rosea: a computer simulation. Bot. Gaz., 145: 184-195, 1984.
7. J.W. Carlyle, S.A. Greibach & A. Paz, A two-dimensional generating system modeling growth by binary cell division. Proc. 15th Annual Symp. on Switching & Automata Theory, New Orleans, pp. 1-12, 1974.
8. J.W. Carlyle, S.A. Greibach & A. Paz, Planar map generation by parallel binary fission/fusion grammars. In: "The Book of L", edited by G. Rozenberg & A. Salomaa, Springer-Verlag, Berlin, pp. 29-43, 1986.
9. K. Culik II & I. Fris, The decidability of the equivalence problem for DOL systems. Inf. and Control, 35: 20-39, 1977.
10. K. Culik II & J. Karhumäki, A new proof for the DOL sequence equivalence problem and its implications. In: "The Book of L", edited by G. Rozenberg & A. Salomaa, Springer-Verlag, Berlin, pp. 63-74, 1986.
11. K. Culik II & A. Lindenmayer, Parallel graph generating and graph recurrence systems for multicellular development. Int. J. Gen. Syst., 3: 53--66, 1976.
12. K. Culik II & D. Wood, A mathematical investigation of propagating graph OL-systems. Inf. and Control, 43: 50-82, 1979.
13. M.J.M. de Boer & A. Lindenmayer, Map OL-systems with edge label control: Comparison of marker and cyclic systems. In: "Graph Grammars and Their Applications to Computer Science, 3rd Int. Workshop", edited by H. Ehrig et al., Lect. Notes in Comp. Sci., in press.
13a M. de Does & A. Lindenmayer, Algorithms for the generation and drawing of maps representing cell clones. In: "Graph Grammars and Their Applications to Computer Science, 2nd Int. Workshop", edited by H. Ehrig et al,, Lect. Notes in Comp. Sci. 153: 39-57, 1983.
13b C.G. de Koster & A. Lindenmayer, Discrete and continuous models for heterocyst differentiation in growing filaments of blue-green bacteria. Manuscript, 1986.
13c P.G. Doucet, The syntactic inference problem for DOL-sequences. In: "L Systems", edited by G. Rozenberg & A. Salomaa, Lect. Notes in Computer Science 15: 146-161, 1974.
14. A. Ehrenfeucht & G. Rozenberg, A limit for sets of subwords in deterministic TOL systems. Inf. Proc. Letters 2: 70-73, 1973.
15. A. Ehrenfeucht & G. Rozenberg, On the subword complexity of locally catenative DOL languages. Inf. Proc. Letters 16: 7-9, 1983.
15a. P. Eichhorst & W. Savitch, Growth functions of stochastic Lindenmayer systems. Information and Control, 45: 217-228, 1980.
16. J.B. Fisher & H. Honda, Computer simulation of branching pattern and geometry in Terminalia (Combretaceae), a tropical tree. Bot. Gaz., 138: 377-384, 1977.
17. D. Frijters, An automata-theoretical model of the vegetative and flowering development of Hieracium murorum L. Biol. Cybernetics, 24: 1-13, 1976.
18. D. Frijters & A. Lindenmayer, A model for the growth and flowering of Aster novae-angliae on the basis of table ⟨1,0⟩ L-systems. In: "L-Systems", edited by G. Rozenberg & A. Salomaa, Lect. Notes in Comp. Sci. 15: 24--52, 1974.
19. D. Frijters & A. Lindenmayer, Developmental descriptions of branching patterns with paracladial relationships. In: "Automata, Languages, Development", edited by A. Lindenmayer & G. Rozenberg, North-Holland Publ. Co., Amsterdam, pp. 57-73, 1976.
20. I. Gnutzmann, Zum syntaktischen Inferenzproblem bei Lindenmayer-Systemen. Dissertation, Univ. Hannover, 1979.
21. F. Hallé, R.A.A. Oldeman & P.B. Tomlinson, "Tropical Trees and Forests, An Architectural Analysis", Springer-Verlag, Berlin, 441 pp, 1978.

21a. C. Harte & A. Lindenmayer, Mitotic index in growing cell populations: Mathematical models and computer simulations. Biol. Zentralblatt, 102: 509-533, 1983.

22. G.T. Herman & G. Rozenberg, "Developmental Systems and Languages". North-Holland Publ. Co., Amsterdam, 363 pp., 1975.

23. G.T. Herman & A. Walker, The syntactic inference problem as applied to biological systems. In: "Machine Intelligence", edited by B. Meltzer & D. Mitchie, Edinburgh Univ. Press, 7: 341-356, 1972.

24. G.T. Herman & A. Walker, Context-free languages in biological systems. Int. J. Comp. Math. 4: 369-391, 1975.

25. P. Hogeweg & B. Hesper, A model study of biomorphological description. Pattern Recognition, 6: 165-179, 1974.

26. H. Honda, Description of the form of trees by the parameters of the tree--like body: effects of the branching angle and the branch length on the shape of the tree-like body. J. Theor. Biol., 31: 331-338, 1971.

27. H. Honda, P.B. Tomlinson & J.B. Fisher, Two geometrical models of branching of botanical trees. Annals of Botany, 49: 1-11, 1982.

28. J.E. Hopcroft & J.D. Ullman, "Introduction to Automata Theory, Languages and Computation". Addison-Wesley Publ. Co., Reading, Mass. 418 pp, 1979.

29. J.M. Janssen & A. Lindenmayer, Models for the control of branch positions and flowering sequences of capitula in Mycelis muralis (L.) Dumont (Compositae). New Phytologist, 105: 191-220, 1987.

30. N.D. Jones & S. Skyum, Complexity of some problems concerning L-systems. Math. Systems Theory, 13: 29-43, 1979.

31. N.D. Jones & S. Skyum, A note on the complexity of general DOL membership. SIAM J. Computing, 10: 114-117, 1981.

32. H. Jürgensen, Probabilistic L systems. In: "Automata, Languages, Development", edited by A. Lindenmayer & G. Rozenberg, North-Holland Publ. Co., Amsterdam, pp. 211-225, 1976.

33. H. Jürgensen & A. Lindenmayer, Inference algorithms for developmental systems with cell lineages. Bulletin of Mathematical Biology, 49: 93-123, 1987.

34. H. Jürgensen, D.E. Matthews & D. Wood, Life and death in Markov deterministic tabled OL-systems. Inf. and Control, 48: 80-93, 1981.

35. J. Karhumäki, The Ehrenfeucht conjecture: a compactness claim for finitely generated free monoids. Theor. Comp. Sci., 29: 285-308, 1984.

36. A. Kelemenová, Levels in L-systems. Math. Slovaca, 33: 87-97, 1983.

37. Y. Kobuchi & S.Seki, Decision problems of locally catenative property for DIL systems. Information and Control, 43: 266-279, 1979.

38. A.N. Kolmogorov, Three approaches to the quantitative definition of information. Int. J. Computer Math., 2: 157-168, 1968.

39. A. Lindenmayer, Mathematical models of cellular interactions in development. Parts I and II. J. Theor. Biol. 18: 280-299, 300-315, 1968.

40. A. Lindenmayer, Developmental systems without cellular interactions, their languages and grammars. J. Theor. Biol. 30: 455-484, 1971.

41. A. Lindenmayer, Adding continuous components to L-systems. In: "L Systems", edited by G. Rozenberg & A. Salomaa, Lect. Notes in Computer Science 15: 53-68, 1974.

42. A. Lindenmayer, Developmental systems and languages in their biological context. Chapter contributed to [22], 1975 (this chapter appeared in Russian translation in Kiberneticheskii Sbornik, Nov. Ser., 17: 192-232, 1980).

43. A. Lindenmayer, Developmental algorithms: lineage versus interactive control mechanisms. In: "Developmental Order: Its Origin and Regulation", edited by S. Subtelny & P.B. Green, 40th Symp. Soc. Dev. Biol., Boulder, Alan R. Liss, Inc., New York, pp. 219-245, 1982.

44. A. Lindenmayer, Models for plant tissue development with cell division orientation regulated by preprophase bands of microtubules. Differentiation, 26: 1-10, 1984.

44a A. Lindenmayer, An introduction to parallel map-generating systems. In: "Graph Grammars and Their Applications to Computer Science, 3rd Int. Workshop", edited by H. Ehrig et al., Lect. Notes in Comp. Sci., in press.

45. A. Lindenmayer & K. Culik II, Growing cellular systems: generation of graphs by parallel rewriting. Int. J. Gen. Systems, 5: 45-55, 1979.

46. A. Lindenmayer & G. Rozenberg, Parallel generation of maps: developmental systems for cell layers. In: "Graph Grammars and Their Application to Computer Science and Biology", edited by V. Claus et al., Lect. Notes in Comp. Sci. 73: 301-316, 1979.

47. H.L. Liu & K.S. Fu, Cellwork topology, its network duals and some applications - three-dimensional Karnaugh map and its virtual planar representation. Information Sciences, 24: 93-109, 1981.

48. J. Lück & H.B. Lück, Generation of 3-dimensional plant bodies by double wall map and stereomap systems. In: "Graph Grammars and Their Application to Computer Science, 2nd Int. Workshop", edited by H. Ehrig et al., Lect. Notes in Comp. Sci. 153: 219-231, 1983.

49. J. Lück, A. Lindenmayer & H.B. Lück, Analysis of cell tetrads and clones in meristematic cell layers. Botanical Gazette, in press.

50. J. Mäenpää, G. Rozenberg & A. Salomaa, Bibliography of L-systems. Report No. 81-20, Inst. of Appl. Math. and Comp. Sci., Univ. of Leiden, 1981.

51. R.J. Matela & R. Ransom, A topological model of cell division: structure of the computer program. BioSystems, 18: 65-78, 1985.

52. N. Macdonald, "Trees and Networks in Biological Models", Wiley, New York, 1983.

53. B.H. Mayoh, Multidimensional Lindenmayer organisms. In: "L Systems", edited by G. Rozenberg & A. Salomaa, Lect. Notes in Comp. Sci., 15: 302-326, 1974.

54. G.J. Mitchison & M. Wilcox, Rule governing cell division in Anabaena. Nature, 239: 110-111, 1972.

55. M. Nagl, "Graph-Grammatiken, Theorie, Implementierung, Anwendungen", Vieweg, Braunschweig, 375 pp., 1979.

56. A. Nakamura & K. Aizawa, A relationship between graph L-systems and picture languages, Theoret. Comp. Sci., 24: 161-177, 1983

57. A. Nakamura, A. Lindenmayer & K. Aizawa, Some systems for map generation. In: "The Book of L", edited by G. Rozenberg & A. Salomaa, Springer-Verlag, Berlin, pp. 323-332, 1986.

58. A. Nakamura, A. Lindenmayer & K. Aizawa, Map OL systems with markers. In: "Graph Grammars and Their Applications to Computer Science, 3rd Int. Workshop", edited by H. Ehrig et al., Lect. Notes in Comp. Sci., in press.

59. J. van Neumann, "Theory of Self-Reproducing Automata", edited by A.W. Burks, Univ. of Illinois Press, Urbana, 1966.

60. T. Nishida, KOL-system simulating almost but not exactly the same development - the case of Japanese cypress. Memoirs Fac. Sci., Kyoto Univ., Ser. Bio., 8: 97-122, 1980.

61. A. Paz & A. Salomaa, Integral sequential word functions and growth equivalence of Lindenmayer systems. Inf. and Control, 23: 313-343, 1973.

62. P. Prusinkiewicz, Applications of L-systems to computer imagery. In: "Graph Grammars and Their Applications to Computer Science, 3rd Int. Workshop", edited by H. Ehrig et al., Lect. Notes in Comp. Sci., in press.

63. R. Ransom, Computer analysis of cell division in Drosophila imaginal discs: model revision and extension to simulate leg disc growth. J. Theor. Biol., 66: 361-378, 1977.

64. A. Rosenfeld & J.P. Strong, A grammar for maps. In: "Software Engineering", edited by J. Tou, Academic Press, New York, 2: 227-239, 1971.

65. A. Rosenfeld, Array and web grammars. In: "Automata, Languages, Development, edited by A. Lindenmayer & G. Rozenberg, North-Holland Publ. Co., Amsterdam, pp. 517-529, 1976.

66. G. Rozenberg & P.G. Doucet, On OL languages. Inf. and Control, 19: 302-318, 1971.

67. G. Rozenberg & A. Lindenmayer, Developmental system with locally catenative formulas. Acta Inf., 2: 214-248, 1973.

67a. K. Ruohonen, Developmental systems with interaction and fragmentation, Inf. and Control, 28: 91-112, 1975.

68. G. Rozenberg & A. Salomaa, "The Mathematical Theory of L Systems", Academic Press, New York, 352 pp., 1980.
69. A. Salomaa & M. Soittola, Automata-Theoretical Aspects of Formal Power Series. Springer-Verlag, New York, 171 pp., 1978.
70. U. Schmidt, Syntaktische Inferenz von DTOL-Systemen. Diplomarbeit, T.H. Darmstadt, 1983.
71. A.L. Semenov & V.S. Guba, pers. commun., 1985.
72. P.L.J. Siero, G. Rozenberg & A. Lindenmayer, Cell division patterns: syntactical description and implementation. Computer Graphics and Image Proc., 18: 329-346, 1982.
73. R. Siromoney, G. Siromoney & K. Krithivasan, Array grammars and kolam. Computer Graphics and Image Proc., 4: 63-82, 1974.
74. R. Siromoney, Array languages and Lindenmayer systems - a survey. In: "The Book of L", edited by G. Rozenberg & A. Salomaa, Springer-Verlag, Berlin, pp. 413-426, 1986.
75. A.R. Smith III, Introduction to and survey of polyautomata theory. In: "Automata, Languages, Development", edited by A. Lindenmayer & G. Rozenberg, North-Holland Publ. Co., Amsterdam, pp. 405-422, 1976.
76. A.R. Smith, Plants, fractals and formal languages. Computer Graphics, 18(3): 1-10, 1984.
77. A.L. Szilard & R.E. Quinton, An interpretation for DOL systems by computer graphics. Science Terrapin (Univ. of West. Ont.), 4(2): 8-13, 1979.
78. A.H. Veen & A. Lindenmayer, Diffusion mechanism for phyllotaxis. Plant Physiol., 60: 127-139, 1977.
79. P.M.B. Vitányi, "Lindenmayer Systems: Structure, Languages and Growth Functions", Mathematical Centre Tracts, No. 96, Amsterdam, 209 pp., 1980.
80. J. White, editor, "Studies in Plant Demography, A Festschrift for John L. Harper", Academic Press, Orlando, 393 pp., 1985.
81. H. Yamada & S. Amoroso, Structural and behavioural equivalences of tessellation automata. Inf. and Control, 18: 1-31, 1971.

A FORMAL MODEL OF KNOWLEDGE-BASED SYSTEMS
(Extended Abstract)

Ivan Kalaš
Institute of Computer Science, Comenius University
842 43 Bratislava, Czechoslovakia

I. INTRODUCTION

Much effort has been carried out in order to build rather complex programs that are able to perform difficult tasks like trouble-shooting, finding a diagnosis, monitoring a system, etc. These tasks are commonly performed by well educated, trained and experienced people we call experts.

Because large body of domain-specific knowledge is essential in these activities, traditional approaches are not quite sufficient in programming these systems. Therefore a new architecture has been adopted which keeps knowledge apart from both control mechanism and data base.

Computations of knowledge-based systems are realized with respect to the structured contents of their knowledge bases and this is the reason why the notion of **inference** is preferred. Many different representation schemes are used to encode knowledge necessary to fulfil this task. Nevertheless, a wave of experiments places great emphasis on the more **theoretical side of problems**. This is quite necessary for progress and deeper understanding of the **fundamentals of AI** (artificial intelligence). It is obvious now, that only formal theories of knowledge and knowledge representation can provide a platform for dealing with a number of basic features that information in knowledge bases has. Moreover, a comparison of distinct representation schemes could be carried out within a formal system adopted as a formalization of knowledge.

There already exist several research papers - and collections of them - focusing on theoretical side of knowledge representation, such as [4], [2], [8], [3], [6], [1], [7], [9].

Chapter 4

ARTIFICIAL INTELLIGENCE

II. SOWA'S CONCEPTUAL STRUCTURES

In [9] Sowa presents an ambitious attempt to synthesize knowledge representation research, logic, linguistics, and philosophy. He has developed a clean, well-grounded scheme for knowledge representation which is rather interesting - apart from other reasons - in that it seems to be "frame-like" if one prefers frames, "associative-network-like" if one uses networks, and similarly with logic, relational database approach, etc. Moreover, Sowa shows how his notation - called **conceptual graphs** - is useful for natural language processing, database inference, and knowledge engineering.

In our work we have developed a formal model of knowledge-based systems based on conceptual graphs, although we have not included some aspects of Sowa's theory for the present (modal operators, a possibility to label a node of a graph with another graph, etc.). At the other hand we precisely define the semantics of conceptual graphs and thus formalize the process of inference. We have also incorporated procedural knowledge represented by attached functions (often called demons, actors, transitions). These functions form a very important constituent of many representation schemes (frames, object-oriented programming, etc.), however they are seldom included in formal theories of AI.

Our model unifies a lot of important properties of techniques currently used in knowledge-based systems (procedural attachement, knowledge inheritance, a possibility to extend vocabulary by definitions, etc.). We give a formal treatment of concepts like knowledge base, inference, or equivalence of knowledge-based systems.

As far as graphics are becoming the most promising way of communication with knowledge-based systems, the immediate readibility of representation structures would be welcomed. This is true with conceptual graphs: the overall structure and particular relations among concepts are obvious from their graphical notation.

III. SYNTACTICS OF CONCEPTUAL GRAPHS

First we introduce the notion of a conceptual graph (omitting a lot of technical details that we have worked out in [5]), which is a directed, finite, not necessarily connected graph labeled with symbols of a vocabulary **S**. Conceptual graphs state interrelations and dependences among concepts of a domain.

A **vocabulary** is a 6-tuple $\mathbf{S} = (v, K, \mathbf{R}, \mathbf{Neg}, \mathbf{F}, \leqslant)$ such that:

- v is a set of individual variables $v_0, v_1, v_2, \ldots,$
- K is a set of conceptual symbols, partially ordered by $\leqslant$,
- **R**, **Neg**, and **F** are functions and
- Dmn**R** is a set of relation symbols. For $R \in \mathrm{Dmn}\mathbf{R}$, $\mathbf{R}(R)$ - a **type** of R - is a finite non-empty sequence $(k_0, \ldots, k_{n-1})$ of conceptual symbols,
- similarly each function symbol f from Dmn**F** has a type $\mathbf{F}(f) = (k_0, \ldots, k_{n-1})$ of conceptual symbols,
- $\mathrm{Dmn}\mathbf{Neg} \subseteq \mathrm{Dmn}\mathbf{R}$, **Neg** is one-one and for $R \in \mathrm{Dmn}\mathbf{Neg}$, $\mathbf{Neg}(R)$ is a new symbol $\neg R$ of the same type as R.

A **graph in S** is a 4-tuple $u = (N_u, E_u, f_u, g_u)$, where (N_u, E_u) is a finite, directed graph, f_u is a function from N_u into the set of symbols of **S** (i.e. into $v \cup K \cup \mathrm{Dmn}\mathbf{R} \cup \mathrm{Rng}\mathbf{Neg} \cup \mathrm{Dmn}\mathbf{F}$), g_u is a function from E_u into the set of natural numbers.

If p is a node of a graph u and p is labeled with a variable, we call it a variable node. If p is labeled with a conceptual symbol, we call it a conceptual node. A conceptual node which has no adjacent variable node is called an existential node. If o,p are nodes of u, o is a variable node labeled with v_{i_j} and p is a conceptual node, then we say that v_{i_j} is attached to p.

We define three operations on graphs: P1 (restricting a concept, i.e. replacing a conceptual symbol with one of its subsymbols - in accordance with partial ordering of K), P2 (leaving out a variable node and an incident edge), and P3 (joining two graphs by merging all identically labeled conceptual nodes that have in both graphs the same variable attached to them).

We characterize a set of elementary, **atomic conceptual graphs**: if $v_{i_0}, \ldots, v_{i_{n-1}}$ are pairwise distinct variables of **S**, $R \in \mathrm{Dmn}\mathbf{R}$ is a relation symbol of type $(k_0, \ldots, k_{n-1})$, then

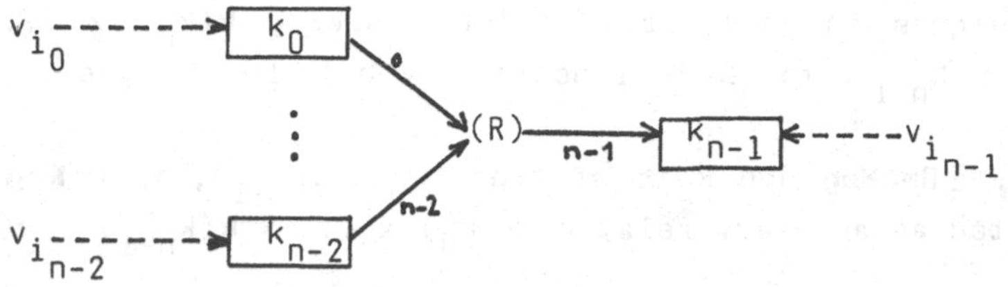

is an *atomic relation conceptual graph*. Similarly we define function atomic graphs and negation atomic graphs for symbols of DmnF and Rng**Neg**. (We draw conceptual symbols in boxes, relation symbols in round brackets and function symbols in diamonds. Edge outgoing from a variable node and edges incoming to or outgoing from a function node are drawn as dotted lines. We omit labeling of edges with natural numbers when not distinctive.)

A set of **conceptual graphs** in **S**, $G_{\mathbf{S}}$, is a set of finite graphs derivable from the set of atomic conceptual graphs by operations P1, P2, and P3. In a natural way we introduce a *derivation* of a conceptual graph. If u is a conceptual graph with variables F(u) = $= \{v_{i_0},..,v_{i_{n-1}}\}$, we let FV(u) be a sequence $\langle v_{i_0},..,v_{i_{n-1}}\rangle$ such that $i_0 < i_1 < \ldots < i_{n-1}$. Conceptual graphs u_0, u_1 are said to be **uniform**, if $F(u_0) = F(u_1)$. u_1 is **subordinate** to u_0, if u_0, u_1 are uniform and for each variable v_{i_j} from $F(u_0)$ it holds: if v_{i_j} is attached to p_0 in u_0 and v_{i_j} is attached to p_1 in u_1, than $f_{u_0}(p_0) \geqslant f_{u_1}(p_1)$, (i.e. label of p_1 is a subsymbol of label of p_0).

IV. SEMANTICS OF CONCEPTUAL GRAPHS

We now introduce the basic notions of the meaning of conceptual graphs. Let **S** be a vocabulary. Then, an **S-structure A** is a 4-tuple **A** = (A,**k**,**r**,**o**), where:

- A is a *domain* over which the variables of **S** can range,
- **k** assignes a meaning to each conceptual symbol of **S**, namely to k it assignes a unary relation **k**(k) on A,
- **r** assignes an n-ary relation $\mathbf{r}(R) \subseteq \mathbf{k}(k_0) \times \ldots \times \mathbf{k}(k_{n-1})$ to each relation symbol R of type $(k_0,..,k_{n-1})$,

- $\mathbf{o}$ assignes an (n-1)-ary function mapping $\mathbf{k}(k_0) \times \ldots \times \mathbf{k}(k_{n-2})$ into $\mathbf{k}(k_{n-1})$ to each function symbol f of type $(k_0,..,k_{n-1})$.

If $R \in \mathrm{Dmn}\mathbf{Neg}$ and R is of type $(k_0,..,k_{n-1})$, then $\mathbf{Neg}(R)$ will be interpreted as an n-ary relation $\mathbf{k}(k_0) \times \ldots \times \mathbf{k}(k_{n-1}) - \mathbf{r}(R)$.

Definition 1: Let $\mathbf{A}$ be an $\mathbf{S}$-structure, $u \in G_{\mathbf{S}}$ be n-ary with $FV(u) = \langle v_{j_0},\ldots,v_{j_{n-1}} \rangle$. Let $a = (a_0,\ldots,a_{n-1}) \in {}^nA$. An **assigment** of a to u is any function $Ass_{a,u}$ from the set of conceptual nodes of u, such that

$$Ass_{a,u}(p) = \begin{cases} a_i & \text{if } v_{j_i} \text{ is attached to p} \\ b \in A & \text{if p is existential.} \end{cases}$$

An assignment $Ass_{a,u}$ **satisfies** u in an $\mathbf{S}$-structure $\mathbf{A}$, if all values assigned to conceptual nodes of u satisfy all relation and function "links" (according to $\mathbf{A}$). Let u be n-ary. A **meaning** of u in $\mathbf{A}$ is a set $u^{\mathbf{A}} \subseteq {}^nA$ such, that $a \in u^{\mathbf{A}}$ if there exists an assignment $Ass_{a,u}$ satisfying u in $\mathbf{A}$.

Two uniform graphs $u_0,u_1 \in G_{\mathbf{S}}$ are said to be **equivalent** in an $\mathbf{S}$-structure $\mathbf{A}$, if $u_0^{\mathbf{A}} = u_1^{\mathbf{A}}$. We say that u_0,u_1 are **logically equivalent** if they are equivalent in every $\mathbf{S}$-structure $\mathbf{A}$.

Theorem 2: It is decidable for arbitrary uniform conceptual graphs u_0,u_1 whether they are logically equivalent.

Example: In an intuitively obvious interpretation the meaning of the following graph consists of all pairs (dog,newspaper) such that there exists a master to whom the dog fetches the daily newspaper in its mouth.

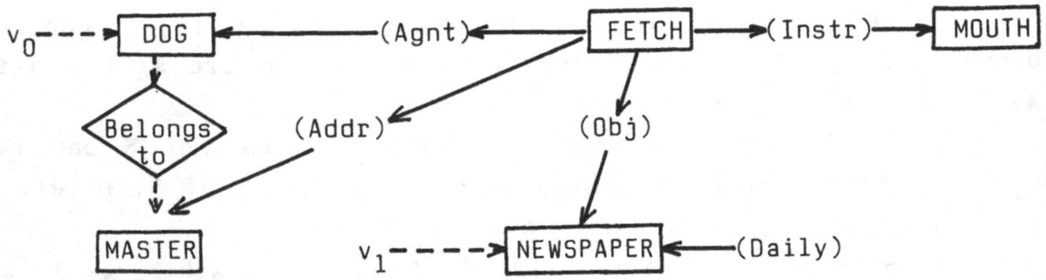

Next we turn to more detailed study of the meaning of conceptual graphs by the meaning of mathematical logic. The role of logic in knowledge representation and reasoning is a lasting issue in AI. However, we believe that this role as a tool for deeper analysis of knowledge is rather important, see e.g. [1]. Logic provides a framework for better understanding the meaning of representation structures, and is a suitable source of referential semantics for them.

We use a kind of many sorted logic with partially ordered set of sorts, to explore correspondence between conceptual graphs and the world. We then prove that the meaning of a conceptual graph is correct (i.e. that it is the same for all derivations of the graph).

Let **S** be a vocabulary. With **S** we associate a many sorted language $\mathbf{L_S}$. For a graph u and its derivation τ we define a **translation** Φ_τ of u, which is a formula $\Phi_\tau(u)$ of $\mathbf{L_S}$. If u is n-ary, then $\Phi_\tau(u)$ has n free variables. Similarly with an **S**-structure **A** we associate an $\mathbf{L_S}$-structure **A'**. By $(\alpha, \mathbf{A}')$ we denote a **meaning** of α in **A'**. The following theorem then holds:

Theorem 3: Let $u \in G_{\mathbf{S}}$, τ be a derivation of u, let **A** be an **S**-structure. Then

$$u^{\mathbf{A}} = (\Phi_\tau(u), \mathbf{A}').$$

Hence it holds that $(\Phi_\tau(u), \mathbf{A}') = (\Phi_\sigma(u), \mathbf{A}')$ for any derivations τ, σ of u.

V. KNOWLEDGE-BASED SYSTEMS

In our model, a domain of discourse is characterized by knowledge encoded in **pairs** of conceptual graphs. Each pair appears as a kind of "substitution rule" in a process of inference. Thus, our formalism parallels the computational architecture of pattern directed inference systems, see e.g. [10].

First we define two kinds of graph operations (omitting some technical details).

- **Subsub(t,u_0,u_1,Z)** - a substitution by subordinate graph - which in a conceptual graph t replaces its subgraph isomorfic with u_0 by u_1, where u_0,u_1 are uniform, u_1 is subordinate to u_0 and a **closure embedding** Z unambiguously determines which subgraph of t is to be replaced,

- **Subinh**$(t,u_0,u_1,Z,(k_0,..,k_{n-1}))$ - a substitution with inheritance - which is more powerful than Subsub. Although u_0,u_1 are once more uniform, there is no subordination required between them. Moreover this operation provides for **knowledge inheritance** by applying rather general piece of knowledge in any specific case (e.g. knowledge concerning all cubes of the "blocks world" may be useful when discussing red cubes supporting blue box B12 in particular). Conceptual symbols $k_0,..,k_{n-1}$ designate these specific concepts under consideration.

An important feature of knowledge-based systems is their continuous incremental growth and the development of specialized technical vocabularies that are used to represent knowledge of the world. This is why we include a mechanism for dynamically defining new concepts and relations among them. The approach is derived from Aristotle's method of definition by "genus and differentiae", see [9], and allows to describe new entities in terms of more primitive ones.

Definitions as well as domain knowledge are encoded in pairs of conceptual graphs, therefore Subsub and Subinh substitutions can be used to introduce **contraction** and **expansion** operations that allow to delete a subgraph and incorporate the equivalent new single concept or relation, and vice versa. Thus moving from new terms to more primitive ones (that define them) and backwards during an inference is possible.

Definition 4: Let **S** be a vocabulary, **A** an **S**-structure. A **knowledge base** B over **A** is a triple B = (**S**, Γ ,D), where Γ is a finite admissible set of definitions and D is a finite subset of the Cartesian product $G_{\mathbf{S}} \times G_{\mathbf{S}}$ such, that (u_0,u_1) in D implies u_0,u_1 are equivalent in **A**. Elements of D are called **domain inference rules**.

The separation of definitions from domain knowledge mirrors two distinct notions of adequacy that a knowledge representation system for expert tasks should address: **terminological adequacy** and **assertional adequacy**, see [3].

The task of a knowledge-based system is to infer the meaning of a stated conceptual graph (which we call question), i.e. to find an appropriate answer.

Procedural semantics provides a procedural acces to only some concepts and relations of the **S**-structure, namely to the meaning of symbols included into a **core** I of the vocabulary **S**. Conceptual graphs labeled only with core symbols are declared **answer graphs**, i.e. graphs with the meaning that can be directly computed in given procedural semantics.

A **knowledge-based system** P over an **S**-structure **A** is a pair P = (B,I) such that B is a knowledge base and I is a core of vocabulary **S**.

An **inference** is an attempt to transform question into an equivalent graph the meaning of which is directly computable. A computational step of this process is provided by an application of a domain inference rule. Beside domain inference rules a collection of **logic**, i.e. universally valid **inference rules**, is also used. Thus, an inference is a search for the conceptual graph's meaning expressed in a procedural, computable way. Definitions and domain knowledge contained in the knowledge base are used to reach that goal.

Next we claim that any inference in P is correct (i.e. the meaning of a question graph is kept throughout the inference):

Theorem 5: Let P = (B,I) is a knowledge-based system over an **S**-structure **A**, let $(t_0,\dots,t_{m-1})$ be an inference in P. Then t_0, t_{m-1} are uniform and equivalent in **A**.

Finally, we define **knowledge** Kn(P) of a knowledge-based system P as a set of all computable conceptual graphs, i.e. graphs for which answers may be infered. Two knowledge-based systems P_0, P_1 are **equivalent**, if they use the same vocabulary, and $Kn(P_0) = Kn(P_1)$.

VI. COMPUTATIONAL POWER OF THE MODEL

As we have seen, there exists a natural mapping of conceptual graphs into the set of many sorted formulas. However, formulas obtained by this mapping are rather simple, so the question of the expressive power of our model is of great interest. We investigate it by means of Turing computability. We show that Turing machines and conceptual knowledge-based systems are - from this point of view - equivalent. Computations of a Turing machine A correspond to inferences of a knowlege-based system P and the next-move-function of A is explicitly represented in the form of domain inference rules.

Given an alphabet Σ, by Σ^+ we denote the set of all nonempty finite words over Σ. We use rather common model of Turing machine $A=(Q, \Sigma, \Gamma, \delta, q_0, q_F)$ with one tape infinite to the right, with the start state q_0 and the final state q_F. By $T(A)$ we denote the set of all words accepted by A, i.e. $T(A)=\{x \mid x \in \Sigma^+ \text{ and } Mq_0 \vdash_A^* q_F M\}$, where $M \in \Gamma$ is a tape symbol marking the leftmost cell and the relation $\vdash_A$ is induced by the next-move-function δ:

$$\delta : (Q - \{q_F\}) \times (\Gamma - \{M\}) \longrightarrow Q \times (\Gamma - \{M\}) \times \{L,R\} .$$

<u>Definition 6</u>: Let Σ be an alphabet, let **S** be a vocabulary. A **coding** (of words by conceptual graphs) is any function c: $\Sigma^+ \longrightarrow G_{\mathbf{S}}$ such that c is recursive and injective.

<u>Theorem 7</u>: There is a coding c such that for any Turing machine A there exists a vocabulary **S**, an **S**-structure **A** and a knowledge-based system P = (B,I) over **A** such that for any $x \in \Sigma^+$:

$$x \in T(A) \iff c(x) \in Kn(P).$$

The coding claimed to exist is defined in such a way, that it visualizes a start instantaneous description of A in the notation of conceptual graphs. Thus, if $x = s_1 \ldots s_n$ is an input word, then c(x) is as follows:

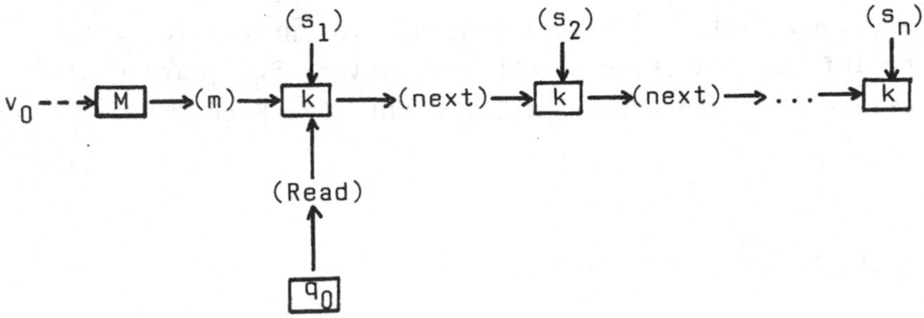

An inference $(u_0, \ldots, u_{m-1})$, where $u_0 = c(x)$, corresponds to an accepting computation $k_0 \vdash_A k_1 \vdash_A \ldots \vdash_A k_{p-1}$, where $k_0 = Mq_0x$. Succesive steps of the inference are determined by the domain and logic inference rules.

There are a lot of quite interesting consequences of theorem 7 - - namely consequences concerning decidability. We will state two of the most important.

Corollary 8: Let P be a knowledge-based system, u a conceptual graph, $u \in G_{\mathbf{S}}$. Then it is undecidable whether u belongs to the knowledge of P.

Corollary 9: It is undecidable for arbitrary knowledge-based systems P_1, P_2 over an **S**-structure **A** whether they are equivalent (i.e. whether $Kn(P_1) = Kn(P_2)$).

VII. SOME COMPLEXITY ASPECTS

Next we investigate some questions concerning complexity of a knowledge-based system. Obviously there are many interesting measures, but so far the size of domain inference rules has been of our main interest. The problem is as follows: Let us suppose there is a knowledge-based system P with one or more "large" domain inference rules. Is it always possible to substitute smaller rules for these large ones so that the resulting system is equivalent to the former system? By a "smaller rule" we understand rule (u_0,u_1) containing conceptual graphs of the size less than a given natural number.

Let us at present consider only **simple** knowledge-based systems, i.e. systems with no definitions (if P=(B,I) and B=(**S**, Γ,D), then $\Gamma = \emptyset$).

By P^+ we will denote a class of all simple knowledge-based systems equivalent to P. So the task is to search P^+ for any Q with "small" enough rules.

Definition 10: Let B=(**S**, Γ ,D) be a knowledge base, let P=(B,I) be a knowledge-based system over an **S**-structure **A**.

(i) a **size** of conceptual graph $u \in G_{\mathbf{S}}$, s(u), is the number of its nodes except those labeled with variables,

(ii) if (u_0,u_1) is a domain inference rule of P, then $\max \{s(u_0), s(u_1)\}$ is a **degree** of (u_0,u_1),

(iii) a **degree** of P, Deg(P), is the maximum degree of all its rules,

(iv) if P is a simple system, then a **minimal degree** of P, $Deg^+(P)$, is $Deg^+(P) = \min_{Q \in P^+} \{Deg(Q)\}$.

Definition 11: Let **S** be a vocabulary. A **rank** of **S** is the maximum rank of its relation and function symbols.

First we investigate the number of simple, nonequivalent knowledge systems, and the number of simple, nonequivalent knowledge-based systems of degrees not greater than k.

To prove resulting proposition 12 we introduce a vocabulary **S**, **S** = (v,K,**R**,**Neg**,**F**,$\leqslant$) with the only conceptual symbol k, two ternary relation symbols +, ., and equality =, and two constants 0,1, i.e. K = $\{k\}$, Dmn**R** = $\{+,.,=\}$, **R**(+) = **R**(.) = (k,k,k), **R**(=) = (k,k), **Neg** = = Ø, and Dmn**F** = $\{0,1\}$, where **F**(0) = **F**(1) = (k).

Let $\mathbf{A}_2$ be an **S**-structure $\mathbf{A}_2 = (A_2,\mathbf{k}_2,\mathbf{r}_2,\mathbf{o}_2)$ such that $(A_2,\mathbf{r}_2(+),\mathbf{r}_2(.))$ is a ring Z_2 of residue classes modulo 2, where $\mathbf{o}_2(0) = 0$, $\mathbf{o}_2(1) = 1$.

We then introduce a class $\{P^2,P^4,P^6,P^8, \ldots\}$ of knowledge-based systems over $\mathbf{A}_2$, P^j being a system corresponding to a commutative ring of characteristic j, and we prove that $P^2,P^4,P^6,P^8,\ldots$ are pairwise nonequivalent. (P^j is a knowledge-based system over $\mathbf{A}_2$, the domain inference rules of which correspond to axioms of commutative ring of characteristic j. That is, if $u \in Kn(P^j)$, then u represents a valid proposition of such rings.)

<u>Lemma 12</u>: There are infinitely many simple, pairwise nonequivalent knowledge-based systems.

<u>Lemma 13</u>: For any given k there are only finitely many simple, pairwise nonequivalent knowledge-based systems of degrees not greater than k.

To prove lemma 13 we define an equivalence relation on a set of all possible inference rules of degrees not greater than k and we show that the number of equivalence classes is finite (in spite of the fact that the number of conceptual graphs of size not greater than k is infinite).

<u>Theorem 14</u>: There is a vocabulary **S** of rank 3 such that for any natural number k there is an **S**-structure **A** and a simple knowledge-based system P over **A** such that

$$\mathrm{Deg}^{+}(P) > k.$$

Proof sketch: Assume the contrary, i.e. for any vocabulary **S** there is such a number k, that for any **S**-structure **A** and simple knowledge-based system P over **A** we have:

$$\mathrm{Deg}^{+}(P) \leqslant k.$$

Let us choose the vocabulary **S** and the **S**-structure $\mathbf{A}_2$ of a ring of residual classes modulo 2. Lemma 13 implies that there are only finitely many simple, nonequivalent systems of degrees not greater than k. As far as any simple system over $\mathbf{A}_2$ is equivalent to one of these finitely many systems, it is in contradiction with lemma 12.

The rank 3 of vocabulary **S** of theorem 14 is not significant. The same statement holds for the rank 2 (which is the least possible rank).

REFERENCES

[1] Bibel, W., Jorrand, Ph. (eds.): Fundamentals of Artificial Intelligence, An Advanced Course, LNCS 232, Springer-Verlag, Paris, pp. 313, 1985

[2] Bobrow, D.G., Collins, A. (eds.): Representation and Understanding, Studies in Cognitive Science, Academic Press, New York 1975

[3] Brachman, R.J., Levesque, H.J.: Competence in Knowledge Representation, Proc. of AAAI'82, pp. 189 - 192, 1982

[4] Hayes, P.: In Defence of Logic, Proc. 5th IJCAI, pp. 559 - 565, 1977

[5] Kalaš, I.: A Formal Treatment of Knowledge-Based Systems, (CSc. dissertation, in Slovak), Institute of Computer Science, Comenius University, 1987

[6] Levesque, H.J.: A Formal Treatment of Incomplete Knowledge Bases, Fairchild Tech. Report No. 614, 1982

[7] Mayoh, B.H.: Unified Theory for Logical Programming and Semantic Representation, Computers and AI 6, No 1, pp. 1 - 15, 1987

[8] Mylopoulos, J : An Overview of Knowledge Representation, in: Proc. of the Workshop on Data Abstraction, Databases and Conceptual Modelling, SIGART Newsletter, No 74, pp. 5 - 12, 1981

[9] Sowa, J.F.: Conceptual Structures: Information Processing in Mind and Machine, Addison-Wesley, pp. 300, 1984

[10] Waterman, D.A., Hayes-Roth, F. (eds.): Pattern Directed Inference Systems, Academic Press, London, 1979

BASIC COMPLEXITY ANALYSIS OF HYPOTHESIS FORMATION

Frederick N. Springsteel
University of Missouri/Columbia
Computer Science Department, Columbia Missouri 65211 USA

1. INTRODUCTION TO GUHA-STYLE HYPOTHESIS FORMATION

Mechanized hypothesis formation of certain general logical forms has been realized in a multilevel system, by the Czechoslovak artificial intelligence project ongoing since 1965, known as the "GUHA Project" [2, 3]. The current overall concept, GUHA-80, is a long-term effort to construct an intelligent analyser of large data sets in the spirit of parallel logic processing [3]. In particular, GUHA-80 applies AI techniques to help expedite data analysis which is "exploratory" (EDA), as opposed to "confirmatory" data analysis. The latter merely confirms a hypothesis once a researcher forms one; the former searches for all patterns, of various types, in the data. MHF as done in the GUHA Circle is necessarily working on an open-ended goal:

> Given large, selected data sets as matrices over a particular domain with dozens of relevant properties as columns and hundreds of observed individuals as rows, the goal is to <u>discover</u> all interesting nontrivial [logical/statistical] implications and/or associations that are plausible hypotheses about the domain, using the properties as unary predicates [2].

"Interesting" is given meaning based on user options but is generally an ill-defined term, as befits an open-ended task. There are copious discussions of this cognitive concept in the GUHA literature [2,3,4,5]. It suffices here to note that it is dealt with in the GUHA-80 project, but we will focus on other aspects. Each GUHA run allows the user to re-define "interesting".

Their current work develops experimental, but key, kernels of the GUHA-80 master plan which in its full extent will be an agenda-driven, rule-based, multilevel AI-system for EDA using parallel processing, with a facet-rich, frame-like knowledge representation structure [3,6]. In many respects its symbolic reasoning is patterned on that of Lenat's AM project [7]. However, EDA deals with real-world empirical data, not pure mathematics. The GUHA-80 system will choose its parallel processes from a wide range of modular algorithms:

- DATA_REDUCTION,

- SIMILARITY_MATRIX,
- CHI_SQuare,
- BMDP3F,
- CLUSTERING (See [3] for a list of GUHA procedures.)

One significant motivation for the overall project is the AI-enhancement of huge statistical software packages, e.g. BMDP, SPSS, SAS, SURVO, etc. [8], for the benefit of ordinary users. These packages are powerful and complex and are somewhat user-oriented, but they usually cannot advise the user about what tool to select from the many possibilities, nor what parameters to use, because there are so many different user situations and variables. Users who are not statisticians, the majority, often need counsel on what software tool should be used in their particular situations.

The first parts of GUHA-80 are approaching this by developing intelligent systems which guide their users in the choice of next procedure to run and its parameters. These new systems draw heavily upon the experience of the expert systems MYCIN and SACON [9,12]. The latter advises users of a multi-part package, MARC. Another AI/analytic system, done within SUMEX, is the RX project, which is like the EMYCIN with the addition of a statistics package [17]; see Figure 1. According to its descriptors, the RX system is admittedly primitive in that it mainly cross-tabulates each domain property versus all others, for significant statistics. It reports very few new results, possibly due to this restriction on form and length of output hypotheses.

2. EXPLORATORY DATA ANALYSIS VIA HYPOTHESIS FORMATION

Recent work on the GUHA-80 objectives has been focused on a prototype expert system, G-QUANT, and on an intelligent multi-statistic evaluator, ASSOC [5]. These kernel procedures deal with (1) the choice of a particular "quantifier", or statistic, from a variety of available modules, and then (2) the detailed evaluation of the chosen statistical or logical formulae over the user's data matrix. There is considerable interfacing between these two modules, and opportunity for positive feedback in their repeated invocation. They form a synergistic pair, like SACON and MARC.

n order to run ASSOC, one must first set the form of quantifier to be sed, e.g. an independence test for two or more properties, like isher's Test, or perhaps one of a class of (non-standard) implications. he expert system G-QUANT serves to help make this choice. Present imlementations utilize six (6) distinct forms, which go way beyond oney-one crosstabs. GUHA hypothesis forms have always been complex enough to relate from two to six different domain properties. Associations of compound (two-way) attributes with a third property are common.

2.1 THE GUHA procedure G-QUANT:

This GUHA module operates more like EMYCIN, without embedded domain knowledge, but with the addition of heuristic rules that give in effect a Logical/statistical Knowledge Base, the expert system G_QUANT; see Figure 2. GUHA runs typically produce much output (unless cleverly restricted), including some novel results [2], but also very many trivial, known or otherwise less interesting hypotheses. G_QUANT was inspired by EMYCIN, as a naked inference engine, but developed independently of it and RX.

The consulting system G-QUANT asks questions of the user like "What is the size of your data matrix?", and then assigns catagories, like "The matrix is: Small/Medium/Large." Then this system employs the technique of backwards chaining, as in SACON and MYCIN, using its knowledge base of heuristic rules of the form:

"IF (condition-1) THEN (condition-2) WITH CERTAINTY (factor)".

Both of condition-i (i=1,2) are true/false propositions related to data analysis, and factor is a knowlege base assigned probability. For example:

> IF (the user wants the results to be decision rules) THEN (the class of the quantifier is IMPLicational) WITH CERTAINTY (1.0);
> IF (the kind of quantifier is Symmetric) AND (the matrix size is Small) THEN (the identity of the quantifier is FISHER) WITH CERTAINTY (0.9);

Actually, to control complexity, G-QUANT does not use a numeric range of "factor" from 0.0 to 1.0, but rather a discrete range of seven values of "c-degrees": from -3 (certainly not) to +3 (certainly yes); 0 means unknown. These c-degrees are assigned to the basic rules, as provided by user evidence, then propagated via the net of rules using the reverse logic of backward chaining, to recommend a quantifier of highest certainty.

2.2 Forming Hypotheses: ASSOC

While this procedure is not an expert system, it is the target of the system G-Quant. ASSOC is a GUHA procedure that processes binary and/or n-ary, i.e. finite-valued nominal data in a "smart" if not intelligent way. It fosters wise choices of input parameters and uses clever default values, to guide novice users. It can also accept real-variable properties and convert them to range-value categories, so that all data is nominal.

ASSOC generates and tests hypotheses. For all six quantifiers these are binary associations of the form:

A ~~S ("A is associated with S")

where A, S are compound propositions for which the atoms are the domain's properties. Non-atomic propositions are formed as disjunctions or conjunctions of signed atoms, and the operator ~~ is to be one of several (generalized) associations, called "quantifiers" [13]. Moreover, conditioned associations of the form (A~~S)/C may be generated as hypotheses, where C is a prior condition for A~~S. Only sentences with disjoint components A, S[, C] will ever be generated; "A" is called the <u>antecedent</u>, "S" the <u>succedent</u>, "C" the <u>condition</u> [14].

In a given run of ASSOC, the quantifier is fixed and so is the condition C (if any); A and S vary. Each generated hypothesis is tested as a statement about the data matrix, by standard methods of evaluation, including cases of missing data. When C is chosen, A~~S is evaluated on the submatrix which omits all rows not satisfying C. If no missing data is detected in the matrix, a proposition pair A,S determines a 4-fold contingency table:

a = # of rows satisfying A & S, |a b|
b = # of rows satisfying A & -S, |c d|
c = # of rows satisfying -A & S,
d = # of rows satisfying -A & -S.

The six quantifiers now used in ASSOC include three symmetric ones:

SIMPLE (association),
FISHER (independence test), and
CHI_SQ(uare statistic),

each of which satisfies a*d > b*c ("coincidence dominates difference"), as well as other defining conditions. The three non-standard, IMPLication quantifiers are:

FIMPL - Founded almost IMPLication,
LIMPL - Lower critical almost IMPLication, and
UIMPL - Upper critical almost IMPLication.

The definitions of these non-standard quantifiers are rather special: for example, (A FIMPL S) is valid iff a > BASE and a/(a+b) > CPROB, given the parameters BASE,CPROB.

Example: Suppose the antecedent A conjoins property #2 and the negation of property #19 and S is property #20 [Suppose these domain properties are respectively: 30-year-chain-smoker, age under 60, and lung cancer]. Then validity holds for

(P2 & -P19) FIMPL P20,

if A is true in 50 rows and both A and S are true in at least 40 of those rows, where BASE = 40 and CPROB = 0.80. In words, the hypothesis: "A 30-year-chain-smoker over 60 is likely to have lung cancer" is true for 80% of the (limited) sample. Matrices with missing data are processed using one of 3 possible semantics: "secured" (the default), "deleting", or "optimistic"; see [13]. These use, instead, a nine-fold contingency table for three-valued logic. Other quantifiers are defined and discussed in [14]. The planned maintenance of the new systems G-QUANT and ASSOC allows for the addition of new quantifiers, as long ad they are "founded" and, preferably, "associational"; see [14]. [The programming for the ASSOC system was done by P. Hajek, I. Hlaveseva, B. Louvar, D. Pokorny, A. Sochorova and E. Tschernoster. The implementation of the G_QUANT expert system was in PL/I, by Marie Hajkova, using IBM 370.]

2.3 Control of Complexity of GUHA/HF Computations

To suppress output of hypotheses implied by already found ones, ASSOC runs use one or both of two logical rules: "Symmetry" for the symmetric quantifiers, and "Improvement" (either "strict" or "conservative") for all six. Improvements of A~~S would only increase its validizing statistics. The need for GUHA processes to preserve strict limits on combinatorial explosion, and principles for doing so, were noted by Springsteel, and by Pudlak & Springsteel [16,15]. Later versions of ASSOC, which will allow more quantifiers, are planned to utilize some of the complexity-induced principles for bounding two-valued logic searches. These principles can best be discussed here in the context of a search for Disjunctions of at most n signed (and distinct) predicates, which disjunctions are to be true for each individual row in the data sample, where n is the total number of atmoic properties. I.e., we assume all basic propositions are in their Disjunctive Normal Forms. We shall denote an instance of this problem by $D_<(M)$, where M is the given mxn data matrix, or simply by $D_<$ for the general algorithmic problem. The first principle allows less output:

EXTENSION: If one disjunction, say d = P1|...|...|Pk, is true in M, then there are at least 2^{n-k} different disjunctions of the maximum length, n, that are true in M. [The latter are the extensions of d by each sign pattern on the (n-k) signed atoms: $(+|-)P_{k+1},\ldots,(+|-)P_n$ Thus, $D_<(M)$ is true if and only if the instance $D_{max}(M)$ is true of maximum length disjunctions. The second principle is:

EXCLUSION: A non-trivial disjunction, d of maximum length n is false over matrix M if and only if the n-tuple of 0's and 1's which negates the Pi's signs is in M.

Thus, $D_{max}(M)$ is true if and only if at least one possible row is missing from M, and a true d can be found by probing for a missing row, linearly. Note that the Principles of Extension and Exclusion imply that not only is D_{max} solvable in polynomial times, over a "search space" of 2^n maximum length disjunctions, but so is $D_<$, over a much larger search space. For example,

d = P1| -P2| P3

is false only when any row <0,1,0,...,...,...> is present in M; this is easily checked. But, if d is thereby found true, so are all extensions of d to maximum length.

2.3.1 Example A: Short Disjunctions Can Play "Hard-to-Get"

Seven people are asked six Y/N questions, including sex (P3, where "1" signifies male), and five either-or preferences. Each person answers independently, but an easy analysis shows there to be several patterns of respones common to all seven. This follows from the Exclusion Principle in general, because 7 is much smaller than $2^n = 2^6 = 64$; thus, many "falsifying rows" must be missing from M. Suppose the responses are:

M: Respondees	Preferences					
	P1	P2	P3	P4	P5	P6
R1	0	0	0	1	1	1
R2	0	0	1	1	1	0
R3	0	1	0	1	0	1
R4	0	1	1	1	0	0
R5	1	0	0	0	1	1
R6	1	0	1	0	1	0
R7	1	1	0	0	0	1

ince 7 is actually less than 2^3, in any 3 columns we can apply Exclu-ion to find true disjunctions of only 3 properties. Using the four ossible sequences of consecutive columns, we can find, in this special ample, exactly one length-three pattern true for every individual and sequence of columns:

-P1|-P2|-P3, -P2|-P3|P4, -P3|P4|P5, P4|P5|P6

The fourth disjunctive pattern here says that everyone answered at least one of the last three questions "Yes". By the Principle of Extension, each of these patterns can be extended arbitrarily by signed predicates that are missing in it, to any length 4, 5, or 6. However, it is not necessary to output these "seen-at-a-glance" consequences of the algorithmically discovered length-3 patterns.

Now, one can try to use Extension to ask if any disjunctions shorter than length three could be true in the M above, meaning length two since no column is all 1's. If any length-2 disjunction were true, it would have two arbitrary extensions of length three using any extra column. By the above results, from an exhaustive search only of consecutive properties, we know that this does not happen for two adjacent columns. Indeed, M contains a full complement of 0's and 1's (four distinct rows) in any pair of adjacent columns! (M is minimal such.)

But how can we know if ANY two columns are full without looking at all pairs? It turns out that we can't in this case, unless we notice that M has "opposite" columns, modulo every third one, e.g., P1 = -P4, etc. Hence, P1 | P4, P2 | P5, and P3 | P6 are true over M, as are the same with all negated predicates. However, in some sense we had to look at arbitrary pairs of the n columns, or "n choose k" combinations, which becomes exponential for k > 2, arbitrary.

2.3.2 Example B: Minimal Seven Rows Without Length-2 Truths

Suppose the survey used above was seen to be concocted, and then refined to ask the same seven people six different 0/1 preferences. Call these changed questions C1 through C6. Answers may be as follows:

M':	Preferences					
Respondees	C1	C2	C3	C4	C5	C6
R1	0	0	0	0	0	0
R2	0	1	0	1	0	1
R3	1	0	1	0	1	0
R4	1	1	1	1	1	1
R5	0	1	1	0	1	1
R6	1	0	1	1	0	1
R7	1	1	0	1	1	0

A perceptive reader (i.e., exploratory data analyst) will realize that some pairs of respondees now fall into patterns like the questions did before: R1 = -R4, R2 = -R3. The latter two responded with opposite "alternate-the-answers" strategies. But this has little to do with finding true length-2 disjunctions, IF any exist. To find the latter, the agent will need to look at each pair of columns, to see if they always agree or always disagree. It turns out that M' has no true length-two's, and seems to be minimally so. For cases like this, it appears "length-k" examples will take exponential time.

It turns out that no length-2 disjunctions are true in M', but clearly many length-3's are, since 7 < 8. E.g., C1|C2|-C3, meaning C3 implies (C1|C2). Thus the design of the new questionnaire is superior: some sample of size 7 (these folks) has no simple pattern of length less than 3 true in M'. [These examples generalize.] Therefore, systems like RX, which seek only length-two valid statements will find nothing true in this M'.

2.3.3 Example C: Truth Comes in All Sizes, Negatively

The previous examples used the fact that with only $n < 2^{n/2}$ rows there must be true disjunctions of length n/2, in ANY n/2 columns of a binary matrix. It is possible with more than $2^{n/2}$ rows that there will still be short, true disjunctions, e.g., some column may be all 1's or all 0's. Thus a matrix with 6 columns and as many as 32 (or, $n^6/2$) rows, the full 5-column binary matrix with an extra columns of 0's, has true disjunctions of ALL lengths, but no purely POSITIVE-predicate disjunctions at all! But, when m increases to at most $16 = 2*2^{n/2}$ rows, we can find special examples, like Example B, with no true length-n/2 formulae. (See [16].)

These examples show the difficulty, and almost the complexity, of the search for true disjunctions in simple two-valued matrices. Other work by this author demonstrates that even very tractable two-valued problems can instantly turn into NP-complete problems when a third logic value is introduced. Also, in general, the problems are harder when the search is for associational quantified hypotheses, but few quantifiers have been studied. Furthermore, certain HF problems seem to fall into natural intermediate complexity classes: their known time bounds are non-polynomial, non-exponential functions such as

$$N^{\log N}.$$

See [16] for a review of these difficulities; it shows the Czechs' limitations on size of desired outputs to be wisely efficient.

2.4 Selected Results in Hypothesis Formation Complexity Analysis

Here we examine certain results concerning the EXISTENCE of desired disjunctive form hypotheses true over given 2-valued (or, 3-valued) data matrices. As above, we shall denote the problem of algorithmically determining whether such hypotheses exist for given conditions by:

Notation Problem [where $\ell(M) = n$, the number of columns]

D_{max} Given any M, is there a maximum length disjunction true in M?

$D_{<}$ Given any M, is there a disjunction of length at most $\ell(M)$ true in M?

D_{par} Given any M and any parameter $k \leq \ell(M)$, is there a disjunction of length k true in M?

$D_{\frac{1}{2}}$ Given any M, is there a disjunction of length at most $\ell(M)/2$, true in M?

These problems can also be posed for Positive disjunctive forms, so denoted by a superscript '+'. We assume all disjunction sought are of elementary form (no predicate occurs twice), all predicates are unary properties and are considered universally quantified (over all rows in the matrices). Obviously, such types of problems include as special cases simple implications:

$$(P1 \mid -P2) \mid P3 \equiv (-P1 \; \& \; P2) \Rightarrow P3.$$

Therefore, even length three disjunctions are of more generality than the problems considered in the RX project.

2.4.1 Two-valued Disjunctive Existence Results

I. D^{+}_{max} is in P; in fact it is solvable in linear time and in log n space.
Proof: There is only one d; test it!
Corollary: $D^{+}_{<}$ is in P.
Proof: Principle of Extension makes these equivalent. [X]

II. D_{max} is in P.
Proof: Use the Principle of Exclusion to probe for any missing row in M, in linear time and logarithmic space. [X]
Corollary: $D_{<}$ is in P, with time and space as above.

III. $D_{\frac{1}{2}}$ is in P. [Modify the proof IV, below.]
Corollary: Given a fixed k, the D_{par} problem is in P.

IV. D_{par} is solvable, all k, in $_N\log N$ time, $(\log N)^2$ space.

Proof: Given M with m rows, and $k \leq n = \ell(M)$, if: (a) $m < 2^k$ then the Exclusion principle produces true disjunctions over any k columns; so, the answer is "Yes"; (b) $M \geq 2^k$, then generate all length-k d's in some numeric order and test on M. The number of such d is at most $(n\ k) * 2^k < (2n)^k = O(_n\log m)$. Say "Yes" if any exist. [X]

[Notice that the median case, $k = \ell(M)/2$, is $D_{\frac{1}{2}}$.]

V. D^+_{par} is NP-complete, as is $D^+_{\frac{1}{2}}$.

Proof: Reduce this one to the NODE_COVER problem; cf. [15].

2.4.2 Three-valued Disjunctive Existence Results

To distinguish these problems from the above two-valued cases where all matrices contain only 0's or 1's, we adjoin an X in the notation. Here the M may contain entries from (0,1,X) where X denotes "unknown". Disjunctions are evaluated on such M by standard 3-valued logic.

I'. D^+_{max} (X) is in P.

(Proof in [15].)

II' - V': The three-valued problems are NP-complete. For example, we demonstrate II'.

Proof of II': $D_{max}(X)$ is isomorphic to the originally proven NP-complete problem SATISfaction of boolean CNF's, $F = \&(C_i)$, over n atomic variables (1,2,...,n) and their negations, per the Reduction:

Suppose F has m clauses. Transform F to the mxn 3-valued matrix M where M(i,j) is: 1 if clause C_i contains variable j, 0 if C_i contains -j, and X otherwise.

It can be checked that a truth assignment to (1,2, ...,n) satisfying F corresponds to one set of signs on properties (columns) P1,P2,...,Pn yielding a true disjunction over m, and conversely. The map F→M is log space. [X].

Most of the positive disjunctive forms of III' -V' follow from reductions to the NODE_COVER problem, via the previously seen NP-complete D^+_{par} two-valued case, as shown in [15].

2.5 ASSOCIATIONAL HYPOTHESES EXISTENCE RESULTS

These problems will be denoted by "A" in place of "D", even though we still assume that the two sides of the associations are each in boolean disjunctive form: ~ denotes (simple) association.

$A_{max}+$: Given any M over (0,1), are there positive disjunctions d, d' of total length $\ell(M)$ such that d~d' is true in M?

[It is an Open Problem where the above set fits in the hierarchy!] Likewise, $A_{max}(X)$ denotes the same problem for arbitrary disjunctions d, d', but over three-valued M.

2.5.1. Two-valued Associational Results

P-time solvable: A_{max}; $A_{<}$; $A_{\frac{1}{2}}$.
N^{logN} solvable: A_{par}.
OPEN PROBLEMS: A^{+}_{par} and all such Positive cases.

2.5.2 Three-valued Associational Problems

We define here a special-form positive-parts associational problem that, as an exception, has a P-time solution. All other cognates of the above problems have been shown to be NP-complete. (See Table 1.)

$A^{+}_{max-1}(X)$: Given any M over (0,1,X), are there positive disjunctions d, d' of lengths m-1, 1 respec., such that d~d' is true in M?

Proposition: The above problem is solvable in linear time.
Proof: The possible choices for d', hence d, are linear in $\ell(M)$. [X]
The above proposition gives hope to the practical side of GUHA-style research, because almost all important (e.g., medical) questions are phrased in terms of what combination of subject properties associate with one specific property, e.g., disease. Similar considerations make disjunctive problems important to finding what implications from a conjunctive (negated premiss) combination of properties, or lack thereof, yield one highly interesting conclusion. There are as yet few results on other quantifiers, e.g. Chi-SQuare ($\sim^2$). One negative result appearing in the appendix of [15] shows that all the $\sim^2$ three-valued problems are NP-complete.

OPEN QUESTION: Is D_{par} or A_{par} actually in P-Time? I.e., can the critical subcase for $2^k \leq m < 2^{n/2}$ solved in time less than the exhaustion method's $n^{\log m}$? If so, such a P-time algorithm could conceivably be useful to design an MHF process to decide D_{par} for arbitrary matrices with a moderate number of rows compared to 2^n, but more than 2^k, making the Principle of Exclusion inapplicable.

GENERAL SOLUTIONS: All of the above problems have considered only existential questions, e.g. of whether there exist true length-n or -k disjunctions for the given M. This is a good prior problem to solve before running any GUHA algorithm, for if no output is to result, it would run exceedingly long to discover this! Still, given some tractably solvable existential situation, how do we convert this to knowledge useful in generating ALL the desired interesting hypotheses, as required by the General Goal? As seen in [16], most of these so-called "General" problems are NP-hard!

Heuristic Case I: If $2^k \leq m < 2^{n/2}$, THEN we need not generate all 2^n-m true length-n disjunctions by Exclusion; it suffices to find (some of) their minimal-length representatives, using the following heuristic, where m is approximated by 2^k:
Each length-k reprensentative extends to 2^{n-k} length-n d's, thus the total number of the latter is represented by at most

$$[2^n - 2^k]/2^{n-k} = 2^k - f < 2^k$$

distance length-k true disjunctions, where f < 1. This assumes few short d's extend to equal length-n's, which is not always true! However, each longer one can stand for its many shorter representatives, if necessary, and at most one should generate about m "independent" disjunctions, giving a linear bound.

Cf. Example A.

Heuristic Case II: If $m < 2^k$ and k = n/2, as in Example B, THEN we can generate true length-k disjunctions using ANY k columns for a total possible number of (n"choose"k)*(2^k-m) length-k's, each of which extends to 2^{n-k} length-n's, for a grand product >> 2^n - m, the distinct disjunctions! Thus, here again, as each length-n true disjunction may be the extension of many, many length-k's, we should use the former to keep track of the latter ones and of independence. For example, M' can have at least (6 3) = 20 length-3 truths, but each of them pairs with its complementary columns in one of the 57 length-6 truths.

. EXPECTED FUTURE DEVELOPMENTS IN GUHA-STYLE EDA/MHF

Future EDA/MHF software can benefit from the experience gained in developing the earlier GUHA algorithms, and in the advanced analysis of possible heuristic algorithms. Eventually, when Automated EDA is applied to very large domains and/or data "samples", like a large city's census, it will require a CPU on the order of today's supercomputers, in order to generate all "interesting" basic rules (even of restricted forms) about the city's population. For example, many different types of economic analysis questions could be ansered simultaneously, without each being explicitly asked!

3.1 WHERE WE ARE/Current limitations on automated discovery:

The major limiting factor is the high cost of discovery compared to conventional methods of doing research; specially built systems cost more than people, at least at first. However, IF vital results were discovered this way that were not seeable another way, then the value of EDA systems would be apparent, regardless of cost. It is doubtful that this can be demonstrated soon, only a relative speed of examination compared to humans.

Costs are high because:

(1) collecting and storing data is costly;
(2) building suitable (initial) KB's is expensive (EDA can help later);
(3) processing very large data sets, using the twin KB's to find new knowledge could be very expensive (supercomputers will be justified);
(4) it is inherently costly to extract just the valid AND new hypotheses from all those generable by the system.

3.2 WHERE WE WOULD LIKE TO BE:

The G_QUANT and ASSOC systems increase our understanding of what the larger package should do, and how to do it. Also, the smaller systems could be used directly by an implementation of GUHA-80, as modules. The GUHA approach to EDA seems much in need of a normal-sized expert system for its users, partly because it is non-standard in some sense: GUHA is oriented mainly to nominal data and its procedures tend to generate plausible domain hypotheses, rather than confirming some user-posited hypotheses.

Special features of a newly proposed ("GUHA-90", below) project also make it possible for an applied EDA system to be of benefit to AI. Having large empirical data, one could process them by ASSOC with an implicational quantifier in order to obtain rules of the form:

IF (condition) THEM (conclusion) WITH
CERTAINTY (c-degree).

Such rules form part of the knowledge base in most expert systems.

Thus, it is conceivable that GUHA-90 could be useful to opening the bottleneck of the knowledge Acquisition Problem that every knowledge engineer faces when building a knowledge base from the utterances of human experts. In the spirit of automated research, inspired by Tukey's exploratory data analysis, one aim of this rest-of-century project is to partially automate, and thereby speed up, the abstraction of heuristic KB rules, directly from the data as much as possible. However, this idea needs much research and testing, to test its feasibility further.

3.3 WHERE WE CAN GO/HOW TO GET THERE:

The MOST interesting developments are expected to occur when we combine the best of both (GUHA and RX) worlds: by interfacing a domain-dependent KB with a domain-independent logico-statistics KB having the power of GUHA's general logic system, plus its multi-statistics evaluations. [See FIGURE 3.] This future system will have five major software components:

(1) The Domain-expert KB (DKB), preferably medical for comparisons;
(2) The Logic KB (LKB), much more powerful than RX's one-on-one;
(3) The domain-dependent database (PDB), for patient studies;
(4) The statistics applications system, here called SAS; and
(5) The control system that includes an automatic hypothesis acquirer (AHA), to coordinate the parallel workings of LKB and DKB and to enlarge (occasionally) the DKB.

It seems clear that American implementations of EDA expert systems should not repeat the FORTRAN and PL/I experimental work of the Czechs. In fact, in order to handle the backword-chaining logic and rich knowledge representation framework envisaged for GUHA-80's unmet goals, several types of modern software support must be arranged:

(1) UNIX/C for a productivity-enhancing operating environment;
(2) PROLOG for the AI aspects just mentioned, requiring Logic Programming;
(3) Compiling facilities, for calling SAS from within PROLOG;
(4) Test Advisor module fully integrated into the Evaluation Stat-Package (ESP);
(5) Artificial Hypothesis Acquirer, transforming output hypotheses, after confirmation, into domain rules for the Knowledge Base.
[Note that "AHA" here implies human-interfaced knowledge acquisition!]

Desirable hardware: powerful, multi-station, number crunching superminicomputer with massive disk storage. Medium-to-high resolution graphics, for displays, would be an extra advantage. [While Tukey's version of EDA is more visually oriented, our system will NOT try to do cluster analysis graphically!]

AUTHOR'S NOTE: While such large research projects are inherently expensive, it seems that the most advanced nation should be able to cooperate with one of the smallest in Eastern Europe, in order to effect very state-of-the-art information extraction systems. Consider the gains:

(1) The RX system output is too restricted; it is domain-dependent;

(2) The GUHA system output is too prolific; it is domain-independent;

(3) The combined, binational system could use the best of both present systems: domain KB for soundness and selectivity of results, and the uniquely powerful logic KB of GUHA-90 to increase the likelihood of discovering varied, new and significant results.

ACKNOWLEDGEMENTS: I need to thank profusely my Czech friends and colleagues, mainly contacted through Dr. Petr Hájek in Prague, for the continuing inspiration that their dedication provides. Many of the complexity results herein were the work of P. Pudlák.

I also acknowledge the partial support of National Science Foundation's Information Science Program, grant IST #8503082, which currently supports my research into logical database design.

REFERENCES

1. Tukey J.W., Exploratory Data Analysis, Addison-Wesley, 1977.
2. Hajek P., Havranek T., Mechanizing Hypothesis Formation: mathematical foundations for a general theory, Springer-Verlag, 1978.
3. Hajek P., Havranek T. GUHA-80: an application of AI to data analysis, Computers and Artificial Intelligence 1(1982), 107-134.
4. Hajek P., Applying AI to Data Analysis, Proc. Eurpn. Conf. on AI, Orsay France, 1982, 149-150.
5. Hajek P., Combining functions for certainty degrees in consulting systems, Intl. J. Man-Machine Studies 22(1985), 59-76.
6. Barr A., Feigenbaum E. (eds.), The Handbook of AI, Chapter III: Knowledge Representation, pp. 141-222.
7. Lenat D., AM - an AI approach to discovery in mathematics STAN-CS-76-570, Stanford Computer Science Department 1976.

8. Dixon J. (ed.), BMDP - Biomedical Computer Programs, Univ. of California Press, Los Angeles 1975.

9. Shortliffe E., Computer-based medical consultations: MYCIN, American Elsevier, New York 1976.

10. van Melle W., A domain-independent system that aids in constructing knowledge-based consulting programs, STAN-CS-80-820, Stanford Computer Science Department 1980.

11. Hart P., Duda R., Einaudi M., PROSPECTOR - a computer-based consulting system for mineral exploration, Math. Geology 10, (1978) 589-610.

12. Bennet J., Croary L., Engelmore R., Melosh R., SACON - a knowedge based consultant for structural analysis, STAN-CS-78-699, Stanford Computer Science Department 1978.

13. Hajek P., Havranek T., The new version of the GUHA-Procedure ASSOC: brief description and user's manual, Math. Inst. Tech. Report 1984-#8, Czechoslovakian Academy of Sciences, Prague 1984.

14. Hajek P., The New Version of GUHA Procedure ASSOC - mathematical foundations, Proc. COMPSTAT 1984, Physica-Verlag, Vienna 1984, 360-365.

15. Pudlak P., Springsteel F., Complexity in Mechanized Hypothesis Formation, Theoretical Computer Science 3 (1979), 203-225.

16. Springsteel F., Complexity of hypothesis inference problems, Int. J. Man-Machine Studies 15 (1981), 319-332.

17. Blum R., Discovery, Confirmation and Incorporation of Causal Relationships from a large Time-oriented clinical data base, Computers and Biomedical Research 15 (1982), 164-187.

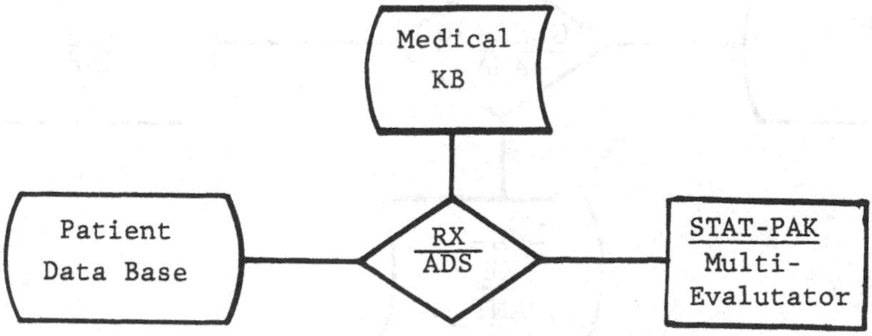

Figure 1. RX Project's Automated Discovery System

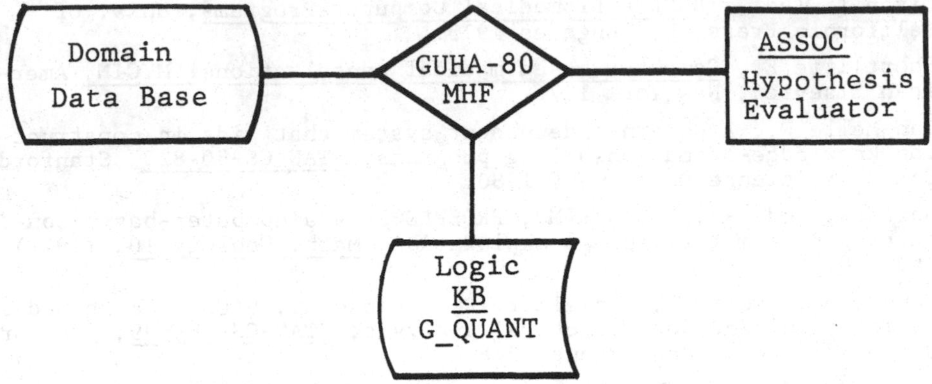

Figure 2. GUHA-80's Mechanized Hypothesis Formation

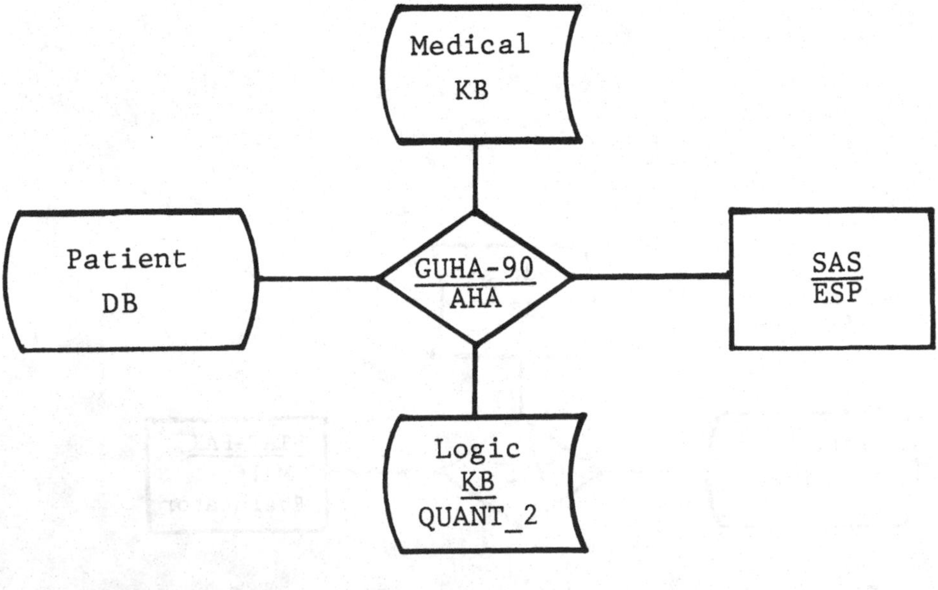

Figure 3. GUHA-90's Artificial Hypothesis Acquirer

Table 1. Reductions for NP-complete Problems

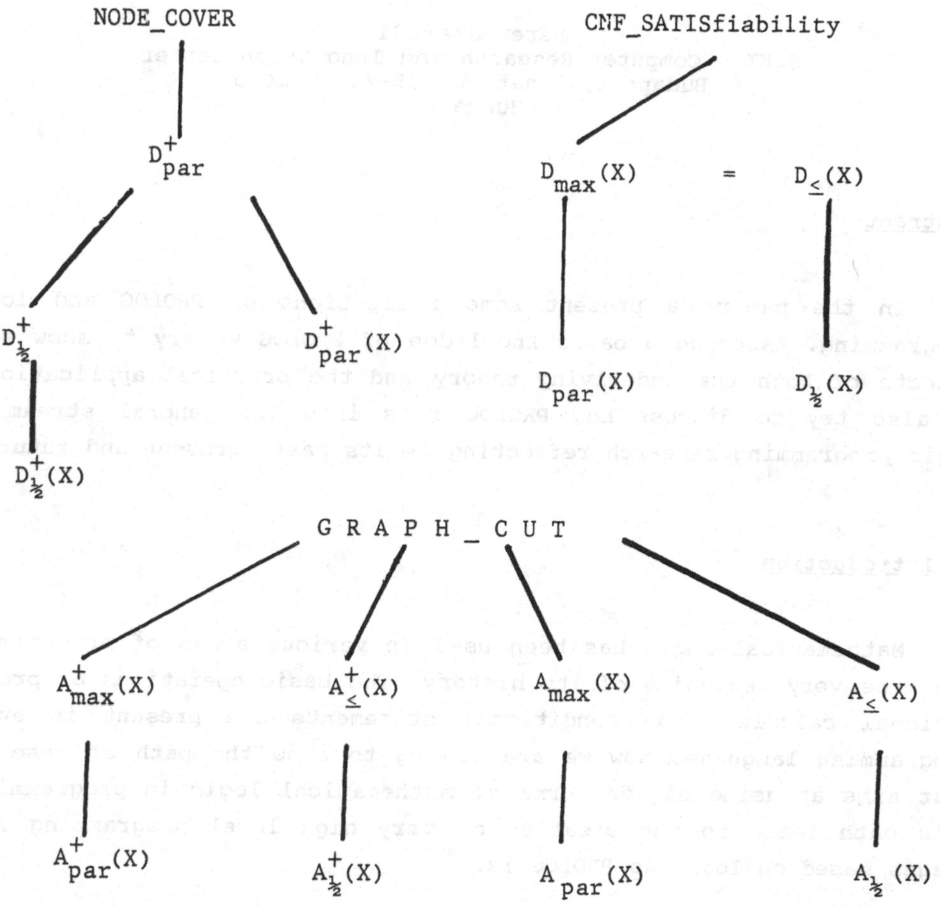

Table 2. Summary of Known Results
[? = unknown complexity]

Type:	2-valued		3-valued	
Restrictions:	D	A	D	A
par	$n^{\log m}$	$n^{\log m}$	NP-complete	
½	P	P	NP-complete	
max	P	P	NP-complete	
≤	P	P	NP-complete	
[positives]	D^+	A^+	D^+	A^+
par	NP-compl.	?	NP-complete	
½	NP-compl.	?	NP-complete	
max	P	?	P	NP-compl.
≤	P	?	P	NP-compl.

PERSPECTIVES OF LOGIC PROGRAMMING

Péter Szeredi
SzKI - Computer Research and Innovation Center
Budapest, Donáti u. 35-45. H-1015
Hungary

Abstract

In the paper we present some reflections on PROLOG and logic programming. Assuming a basic knowledge of PROLOG we try to show some aspects of both the underlying theory and the practical applications. We also try to discuss how PROLOG fits into the general stream of logic programming research reflecting on its past, present and future.

1. Introduction

Mathematical logic has been used in various areas of programming from the very beginning of its history. The basic operations of propositional calculus, the conditional statements are present in every programming language. Now we are trying to show the path of research that aims at using higher forms of mathematical logic in programming. This path leads to the creation of very high level programming languages based on logic as PROLOG is.

In point 2. some aspects of verification and program synthesis systems are discussed and the general principles of logic programming are introduced. In points 3. and 4. features of the PROLOG language are described - its relation to logic programming and also its usability in practical programming. Finally in point 5. current trends of research and development of logic programming and PROLOG are investigated.

2. From "logic in programming" to "logic programming"

Higher forms of mathematical logic, e.g. the first order predicate calculus were started to be used in programming in the early sixties. One of the research directions for facing the software crisis advocated the use of program specifications formulated in mathematical logic to provide safer and more productive software systems. On the other hand various mechanical theorem proving techniques were developed that could serve as tools for implementing such logic based systems.

The first approaches that used program specifications in logic were program verification and program synthesis systems [8]. Let us examine a much simplified schema of these systems as presented in Figs.1. and 2. In a program verification system the user has to supply a program (generally written in some high level algorithmic language) together with a specification in logic of what the given program is intended to do. The verifier uses theorem proving techniques to compare the program and the specification and returns a yes/no answer whether the program is correct with respect to the given specification or not. The process of verification can be performed independently of the actual execution of the program as depicted on Fig.1.

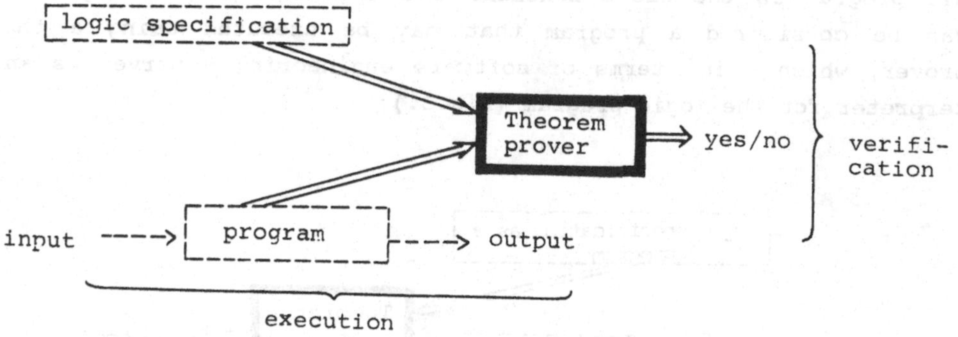

Fig.1. Schema of a program verification system

A program synthesis system takes a logic specification of a program as input and - again using theorem proving techniques - produces a program conforming to the specification (Fig.2.). Of course program synthesis needs more powerful theorem proving techniques than verification in order to <u>construct</u> an executable program. This program can be subsequently executed in the same way as hand written programs.

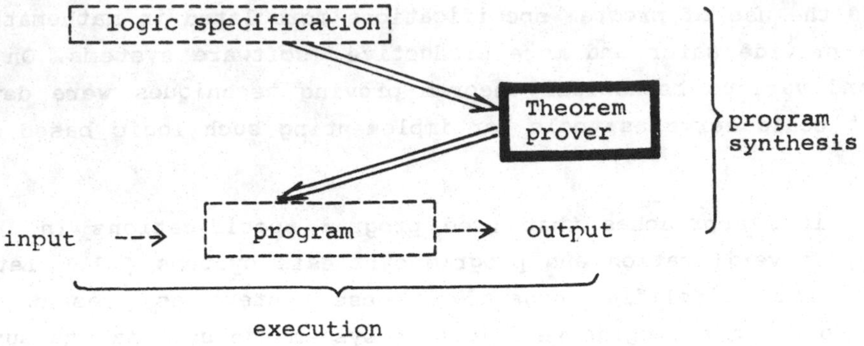

Fig.2. Schema of a program synthesis system

Experience and the problems of theorem provers, verification and synthesis systems all contributed to the appearance of a new research direction: logic programming pioneered by A.Colmerauer, P.Hayes and R.Kowalski in the early seventies [4], [6]. The basic idea of this approach is that one can totally get rid of the "traditional" algorithmic program in the above schemes. The specification in logic itself can be considered a program that may be executed using a theorem prover, which - in terms of software engineering - serves as an interpreter for the logic program (Fig.3.):

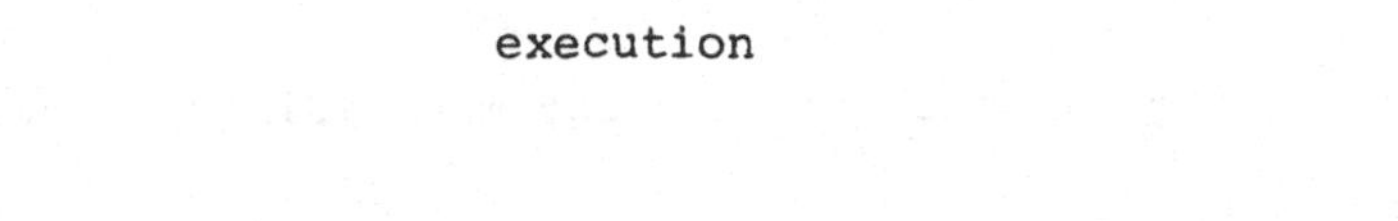

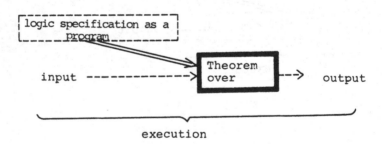

Fig.3. Schema of a logic programming system

Let us clarify the basic idea of logic programming. A logic specification can be thought of as a formula relating the input values $\underline{x}$ of a program to the output values $\underline{y}$: $\varphi(\underline{x},\underline{y})$. If the specification is satisfiable then for each input there exists at least one set of output values, i.e

$$\forall \underline{x} \exists \underline{y}\ \varphi(\underline{x},\underline{y})$$

holds. (We are simplifying the discussion by assuming that the program should work for all input values. It is left to the reader to consider the case when the program and so the formula 'φ' is defined only for input values satisfying some condition '$\psi(\underline{x})$'.) Given now a concrete input $\underline{a}$ one can supply the true closed formula

$$\exists \underline{y}\ \varphi(\underline{a},\underline{y})$$

to a theorem prover which should be able to prove it. If the theorem proving technique is constructive, i.e. an existentially quantified formula is proved by finding a concrete object for which the formula holds, then proving the above formula means constructing a concrete $\underline{b}$ for which

$$\varphi(\underline{a},\underline{b})$$

holds. That means that the result of the theorem proving process is the desired output $\underline{b}$ of the program.

A logic programming system allows the user to write specifications instead of programs - thus implementing the famous slogan "WHAT rather than HOW". Logic programming systems, however, still inherit the major problem of theorem proving: the peril of combinatorial explosion. Proving a theorem is basically finding a specific path in a tree of possible proofs -which may be a practically impossible task if the tree is big enough. There are a number of concepts left open in the general schema of logic programming: the logic language, the theorem proving method and also the strategy of the theorem prover. An appropriate choice of these concepts can help in overcoming the problems of combinatorial explosion.

3. From logic programming to PROLOG

The programming language PROLOG (PROgramming in LOGic) was created in the early seventies at the University of Marseille [12], virtually in parallel with the construction of the theory of logic programming.

As mentioned previously some compromises had to be made in designing PROLOG to avoid combinatorial problems. The first of these was to restrict the language to so called Horn clauses, i.e. statements of form

$$A \text{ if } C_1 \text{ and} \ldots \text{ and } C_n \quad n>=0 \qquad (*)$$

where A and C_k are atomic relations having constants, variables and functional expressions as arguments. Functional expressions consist of a function name applied to a number of arguments of similar form. (*) is usually called a _rule_ if n>0 and an _assertion_ or _fact_ if n=0. All variables in the statement are universally quantified. Note that for variables which occur only in conditions C_k this is equivalent to being existentially quantified within the conditions part:

$$A \text{ if}(\exists \underline{v}(C_1 \text{ and} \ldots \text{ and } C_n))$$

In addition to a number of statements of form (*) one can specify a goal statement

$$C_1 \text{ and } \ldots \text{ and } C_n$$

to be proved.

The theorem proving technique chosen for PROLOG is _resolution_ developed by J.A. Robinson in 1965 [11]. This is one of the most powerful theorem proving techniques, it works on the _clausal form_ of first order logic (of which the Horn clauses are a subset). Its basic operation is unification - a generalization of pattern matching which is used to create the least specialized common form of two atomic relation expressions by substituting variables in both of them.

A number of specialized strategies have been developed for resolution theorem proving. PROLOG uses a form of linear resolution: SL resolution [5]. In addition to that, most common PROLOG implementations apply strict selection rules in traversing the search tree of proofs. This results in a very simple proof strategy that can also be described in more traditional terms of pattern directed procedure invocation and backtracking, leading to procedural semantics which is used in most PROLOG textbooks, e.g. [2].

On approaching PROLOG from the theorem proving side one can be seriously disappointed. The restriction to Horn clauses means that one can not use negation, implication or universal quantifiers in the conditions of a rule. Consequently many relations need to be defined recursively, when one could get away without recursion in full first order logic. An example of this is the relation 'all elements of a given list are positive' which could be something like

```
all_elements_positive(L) if
        (∀X) (member(X,L) implies X>0).
```

in full first order logic. In PROLOG one needs to transform the above to the following:

```
all_elements_positive ([]).
all_elements_positive ([X|L]) if
            X>0 and all_elements_positive(L).
```

PROLOG programs are also especially vulnerable to ordering of statements or ordering of the conditions of a rule. For example the 'ancestor_of' relation can be simply defined by a recursion on the 'parent_of' relation:

```
A ancestor_of D if A parent of D.
A ancestor_of D if A parent_of C and C ancestor_of D.
```

If we exchange the order of the two conditions in the second statement the PROLOG execution mechanism will enumerate all ancestors and then loop. If in addition we exchange the two statements then PROLOG will loop immediately.

If, however, one looks at PROLOG as a programming language it shows a number of high level features. The most important of these are the following

a. Double semantics - in addition to procedural semantics PROLOG statements have a well defined meaning in logic: a declarative semantics.

b. Multi-purpose definitions - a relation represents a number of functions depending on which arguments are supplied on invocation and which are not.

c. Backtracking can serve as a high level form of iteration.

d. Unification replaces a number of data handling facilities: selector and constructor functions and also handling of references (pointers)

Let us illustrate the above points on a classical example of list membership

```
member(X,[X|L]).                                        (1)
member(X,[Y|L]) if
          member(X,L).                                  (2)
```

These two statements can be read in a declarative way as follows:

(1) for each X and L a list with head X and tail L has X as its member i.e. a head of a list is its member;

(2) X is a member of a list if it is a member of its tail.

The definition of member can be used for a number of purposes. The simplest use is to check whether a given object is a member of a given list:

```
?- member(3,[1,2,3,4,5]).
```

The answer is: Yes.

It can be used to find a common member of two lists:

```
?- member(X,[1,2,3,4,5]) and
        member (X,[2,4,6,8,10]).
```

The system gives two answers: X=2 and X=4

Here the first call of member chooses an element of the first list while the second one checks whether the selected element is present in the second list. The second invocation of member acts as a filter on the results produced by the first one. This could be implemented by a doubly nested loop in a traditional algorithmic language. Increasing the number of conditions to be satisfied for a given object, corresponds to increasing the depth of nested loops - this shows how enumeration on backtracking in PROLOG replaces complex nested iterations of algorithmic languages.

The same definition of membership can be used to construct a list with given objects as elements. To illustrate this feature we use a more complex data structure for the elements of the list: 'pair(KEY,CONTENTS)'. A list of such pairs can be used to represent a dictionary associating a CONTENTS field with each KEY field. The 'member' predicate can be used both for entering a new pair to the dictionary and for searching a pair with a given KEY field:

```
?- member(pair(a,1),L) and member(pair(b,2),L)
                       and member(pair(b,X),L).

     The answer is: L = [pair(a,1),pair(b,2)|L'']
                    X = 2
```

The first call of member instantiates L to [pair(a,1)|L'], the second one L' to [pair(b,2)|L''] resulting in the above answer. The third call does not instantiate L further, but returns X=2 by matching the given pair(b,X) with the second element at L. Of course, in real applications these calls of member are not consecutive, they are scattered through a recursive program. This example convincingly shows the power of unification replacing complex data manipulation constructs of algorithmic languages.

Summarizing the discussion we have to state that a PROLOG system should not be expected to behave like a general theorem prover. PROLOG should be regarded as a programming language which, however, preserves a number of important features of an ideal logic programming language. For example, in general we cannot <u>write</u> PROLOG programs by describing only WHAT to perform, we do have to consider HOW the program will be executed. The existence of declarative semantics means, however, that a lot of PROLOG programs can be <u>read</u> concentrating on WHAT the program is going to do without paying any attention to HOW this is going to be achieved.

4. From PROLOG to practice

The pure PROLOG language needs to be extended with so called built-in predicates to support "real" programming.

Introduction of some built-in predicate groups - for example of integer arithmetic predicates - do not hurt the basic principles of logic programming. In this case equivalent predicates could be formulated in PROLOG, but the underlying hardware or software can itself perform the necessary operations (e.g. addition or multiplication) so it is worthwhile to allow the PROLOG programmer to access the hardware facilities through built-in predicates. Such built-in predicates can be regarded as relations that are not defined by logical formulae but derive their meaning from some standard model.

Other groups of built in predicates - basically those for input/output - need to be introduced to link the PROLOG system to the usual computing environment. Such predicates can hardly be assigned a declarative reading, their essence is the side effect they produce, but this side effect concerns the external world not the PROLOG system itself.

There are two built-in predicate groups which may cause conflicts with declarative semantics and so give rise to the bulk of controversy: the predicates for controlling the execution and the predicates for program modification (or PROLOG data base handling).

The basic control operation available in all PROLOG implementations is the 'cut' operation denoted by '!' (or sometimes by '/'). One can use the 'cut' just to improve efficiency of the program i.e. to cut out only those branches of the search tree that are known to contain no solutions. This use does not modify the semantics of the program, so the 'cut' can be ignored on declarative reading. The "real" use of the 'cut' is when those branches are cut out which may contain solutions. This is a serious breach of declarative semantics, which, however, can be remedied in certain situations. For example one can give declarative semantics to certain constructs in which 'cut' occurs (switching to a more widespread notation for PROLOG connective ':-' and ',' instead of <u>if</u> and <u>and</u>):

```
d :-
   a, !, b.
d :-
   c.
```

can be read as

```
d if (if a then b else c)
```

or equivalently

```
d if (a implies b and not(a) implies c)
```

provided 'a' is fully instantiated (does not contain free variables) at the moment of execution and also accepting the 'closed world assumption' i.e. that 'not(a)' can be considered true if the proof of 'a' fails.

The program modification predicates are for adding and deleting statements. This of course carries the danger of self modifying programs. The most common use of these built-in predicates is, however, for updating a database of variable-free facts. Even this simple usage is difficult to embed into the theory of logic programming since the modification of a database of facts means changing the axioms during the proof. Let us show a small extension of the "standard" PROLOG predicate set that helps in solving the outlined problem.

In the MPROLOG system ([1] [9]) backtrackable versions of database modification predicates are introduced. With these predicates the change performed on the database is undone when control backtracks over the predicate causing the change. This means that if several alternative branches can be selected at a given point of execution the data base will be restored to the original state before trying a next alternative.

The backtrackable versions of the data base modification predicates are much more clear from the theoretical point of view than the non-backtrackable ones. In fact, the solution proposed by R. Kowalski [7] to overcome the impurity introduced by a changing data base through meta-level reasoning works only for the backtrackable version. On the other hand backtrackable predicates are very useful in the practice of PROLOG programming. We illustrate this by a small example in MPROLOG.

Let us have an undirected graph represented by a data base of facts of form

edge($point_1$,$point_2$)

Such a fact states that there is an edge from '$point_1$' to '$point_2$'. We define a predicate 'path($point_1$,$point_2$) to mean there is a path from '$point_1$' to '$point_2$':

```
path(X,X).
path(X,Z):-
    del_matching_edge(X,Y),path(Y,Z).

del_matching_edge(X,Y):-
    del_matching_statement_b(edge(X,Y)).
del_matching_edge(X,Y):-
    del_matching_statement_b(edge(Y,X)).
```

Here del_matching_statement_b is the backtrackable predicate to find a statement matching its argument and to delete it. Deletion of the matching fact ensures that each edge is used only once, but if back-tracking steps back over the given choice the deleted fact has to be reinserted into the data base to make possible using the given edge in another selection. Note that in the above example the definition of 'del_matching_statement_b' could be given in terms of the built-in predicate 'del_matching_statement' (equivalent of 'retract' in DEC-10 PROLOG) and 'add_statement' (equivalent of 'assert'):

```
del_matching_statement_b (ST):-
         del_matching_statement(ST).
del_matching_statement_b (ST):-
         add_statement(ST), fail.
```

This definition, however, is not only more expensive in terms of implementation, but it is also vulnerable to any 'cut's - these may cut off the 'add_statement' branch in which case undoing is not performed.

5. Future trends in logic programming

The first, very natural question arising in connection with the future of logic programming is: can one expect new logic programming languages to be created that are completely different from PROLOG?

Recent results of M. Szöts [13] show that a constructive theorem proving technique can be developed only for sublanguages of logic that are equivalent to (some subset of) Horn clauses. By constructivity we mean here that at proving an existentially quantified formula a unique object is being constructed for which the formula holds. This result proves that the language of a logic programming system (as outlined in point 2) must be equivalent or weaker than the language of Horn clauses, which means that the subset of logic chosen for PROLOG was in some sense the "best choice". On the other hand we can still create new logic programming languages as long as the language is transformable to Horn clauses in general terms of logical equivalence. In this sense PROLOG can be regarded as a low level, "machine code" language of logic programming and one can design "higher level" logic programming languages that can be transformed to Horn clauses - just as higher level algorithmic programming languages are transformed into actual machine code.

One important aspect where PROLOG needs to be upgraded to a higher level is organization of loops or more exactly recursion. The restriction to Horn-clauses means that one has to use recursion instead of universal quantification as illustrated in point 3 by the 'all_elements_positive' example. Moreover many PROLOG definitions have to be defined by recursion, e.g. the 'split' predicate used in quicksort:

```
split([H|L],X,[H|L1],L2):-
    H<=X, split(L,X,L1,L2).

split([H|L],X,L1,[H|L2]):-
    H>X, split(L,X,L1,L2).

split([],_,[],[]).
```

could be defined in a "higher level" form by something like

```
split(L,X,L1,L2) if
    L1 = list(H elem L suchthat H <= X) and
    L2 = list(H elem L suchthat H > X).
```

Another possible extension of the PROLOG language is the introduction of data types. This helps in improving the readability of programs and also may contribute to solving "loop" organization problems. A recursive data structure e.g. a binary tree can be traversed in several ways - so the language should enable the user to define the data structures and the traversal algorithms together. The traversal algorithms could be named (e.g. left_to_right_breadth_first) and used in loop (recursion) specifications.

Introduction of data types may also help in improving the speed of code generated from a PROLOG program by a compiler. It is a problem, however, that currently available PROLOG systems offering data types (e.g. TURBO-PROLOG based on work of J.F. Nilsson [10]) pose severe restrictions on important aspects of PROLOG e.g. data base handling and meta-programming.

Let us now briefly tackle the two other components of a logic programming system besides the language: the theorem proving technique and the strategy (execution mechanism). Resolution and especially unification seem to have important advantages over other techniques. An example of very few alternative languages is "LOBO" [3]. "LOBO" has no pattern matching but it allows bounded universal quantifiers resulting in a logic programming language that is nearer to traditional programming and simpler to compile - but one looses quite a few advantages of PROLOG, e.g. those described under b. and d. in point 3.

Many research activities have been devoted to improving the very simple and straightforward execution mechanism of PROLOG. Due to lack of space we just list a few topics:

- intelligent backtracking tries to avoid those branches of the search tree which can not change the subgoal that causes backtracking.
- coroutined execution to allow postponing certain subgoals until e.g. some variables become instantiated.
- concurrent execution that makes possible exploiting parallel hardware.

6. Conclusion

PROLOG has been a compromise between the general aims of logic programming on one side and the capabilities of hardware and the power of implementation techniques on the other side. Recently there have been important developments on this second side: dramatic increase of the computing power of generally available hardware and also notable improvements in the compilation technique of PROLOG (see e.g. [10] and [14]).

This will hopefully contribute both to more widespread use of PROLOG which may become almost a general purpose language like Pascal and also to the development of higher level logic programming languages that may bring the "WHAT rather than HOW" principle nearer to realization.

References

[1] J.Bendl, P.Koves and P.Szeredi: The MPROLOG System; Proceedings of the Logic Programming Workshop, Debrecen, 1980, pp. 201-209.

[2] W.F.Clocksin and C.S.Mellish: Programming in Prolog, Springer-Verlag, 1981.

[3] T.Gergely and M.Szöts: Some features of a new logic programming language; Proc. of Workshop and Conference on Applied AI and Knowledge Based Expert Systems, Ed. P.Revai Univ.of Stockholm, 1985.

[4] P.J.Hayes: Computation and Deduction; Proceedings of Symposium on Mathematical Foundation of Computer Science, High Tatras September 1973, pp.105-117.

[5] R.A.Kowalski and D.Kuehner: Linear resolution with selection function; Artificial Intelligence 2, 1971, pp. 227-260.

[6] R.A.Kowalski: Predicate Logic as Programming Language; Proc. IFIP'74, North Holland Publ. Co., Amsterdam, 1974, pp. 569-574.

[7] R.A.Kowalski: Logic Programming; Proc. IFIP'83 North Holland Publ. Co., Amsterdam, 1983, pp. 133-145.

[8] Z. Manna: Mathematical Theory of Computation; McGraw Hill, New-York, 1974.

[9] MPROLOG Documentation, Release 2.1; Logicware, Toronto; SzKI, Budapest, 1985.

[10] J.F.Nilsson: On the compilation of a Domain Based Prolog; Proc. IFIP'83, North Holland Publ. Co., Amsterdam, 1983, pp. 293-298.

[11] J.A.Robinson: A machine-oriented Logic Based on the Resolution Principle; Journal of ACM 12, pp. 23-41.

[12] Ph.Roussel: PROLOG: Manuel de Reference et d'Utilisation; Grouppe d'Intelligence Artificielle; Université d'Aix-Marseille,Luminy, 1975.

[13] M.Szöts: Logical Foundations of Logic Programming; Thesis, Budapest, 1986.

[14] D.H.D.Warren: An Abstract Prolog Instruction Set; Technical Note 309, SRI International, Oct. 1983.

Vol. 245: H.F. de Groote, Lectures on the Complexity of Bilinear Problems. V, 135 pages. 1987.

Vol. 246: Graph-Theoretic Concepts in Computer Science. Proceedings, 1986. Edited by G. Tinhofer and G. Schmidt. VII, 307 pages. 1987.

Vol. 247: STACS 87. Proceedings, 1987. Edited by F.J. Brandenburg, G. Vidal-Naquet and M. Wirsing. X, 484 pages. 1987.

Vol. 248: Networking in Open Systems. Proceedings, 1986. Edited by G. Müller and R.P. Blanc. VI, 441 pages. 1987.

Vol. 249: TAPSOFT '87. Volume 1. Proceedings, 1987. Edited by H. Ehrig, R. Kowalski, G. Levi and U. Montanari. XIV, 289 pages. 1987.

Vol. 250: TAPSOFT '87. Volume 2. Proceedings, 1987. Edited by H. Ehrig, R. Kowalski, G. Levi and U. Montanari. XIV, 336 pages. 1987.

Vol. 251: V. Akman, Unobstructed Shortest Paths in Polyhedral Environments. VII, 103 pages. 1987.

Vol. 252: VDM '87. VDM – A Formal Method at Work. Proceedings, 1987. Edited by D. Bjørner, C.B. Jones, M. Mac an Airchinnigh and E.J. Neuhold. IX, 422 pages. 1987.

Vol. 253: J.D. Becker, I. Eisele (Eds.), WOPPLOT 86. Parallel Processing: Logic, Organization, and Technology. Proceedings, 1986. V, 226 pages. 1987.

Vol. 254: Petri Nets: Central Models and Their Properties. Advances in Petri Nets 1986, Part I. Proceedings, 1986. Edited by W. Brauer, W. Reisig and G. Rozenberg. X, 480 pages. 1987.

Vol. 255: Petri Nets: Applications and Relationships to Other Models of Concurrency. Advances in Petri Nets 1986, Part II. Proceedings, 1986. Edited by W. Brauer, W. Reisig and G. Rozenberg. X, 516 pages. 1987.

Vol. 256: Rewriting Techniques and Applications. Proceedings, 1987. Edited by P. Lescanne. VI, 285 pages. 1987.

Vol. 257: Database Machine Performance: Modeling Methodologies and Evaluation Strategies. Edited by F. Cesarini and S. Salza. X, 250 pages. 1987.

Vol. 258: PARLE, Parallel Architectures and Languages Europe. Volume I. Proceedings, 1987. Edited by J.W. de Bakker, A.J. Nijman and P.C. Treleaven. XII, 480 pages. 1987.

Vol. 259: PARLE, Parallel Architectures and Languages Europe. Volume II. Proceedings, 1987. Edited by J.W. de Bakker, A.J. Nijman and P.C. Treleaven. XII, 464 pages. 1987.

Vol. 260: D.C. Luckham, F.W. von Henke, B. Krieg-Brückner, O. Owe, ANNA, A Language for Annotating Ada Programs. V, 143 pages. 1987.

Vol. 261: J. Ch. Freytag, Translating Relational Queries into Iterative Programs. XI, 131 pages. 1987.

Vol. 262: A. Burns, A.M. Lister, A.J. Wellings, A Review of Ada Tasking. VIII, 141 pages. 1987.

Vol. 263: A.M. Odlyzko (Ed.), Advances in Cryptology – CRYPTO '86. Proceedings. XI, 489 pages. 1987.

Vol. 264: E. Wada (Ed.), Logic Programming '86. Proceedings, 1986. VI, 179 pages. 1987.

Vol. 265: K.P. Jantke (Ed.), Analogical and Inductive Inference. Proceedings, 1986. VI, 227 pages. 1987.

Vol. 266: G. Rozenberg (Ed.), Advances in Petri Nets 1987. VI, 451 pages. 1987.

Vol. 267: Th. Ottmann (Ed.), Automata, Languages and Programming. Proceedings, 1987. X, 565 pages. 1987.

Vol. 268: P.M. Pardalos, J.B. Rosen, Constrained Global Optimization: Algorithms and Applications. VII, 143 pages. 1987.

Vol. 269: A. Albrecht, H. Jung, K. Mehlhorn (Eds.), Parallel Algorithms and Architectures. Proceedings, 1987. Approx. 205 pages. 1987.

Vol. 270: E. Börger (Ed.), Computation Theory and Logic. IX, 442 pages. 1987.

Vol. 245: H.F. de Groote, Lectures on the Complexity of Bilinear Problems. V, 135 pages. 1987.

Vol. 246: Graph-Theoretic Concepts in Computer Science. Proceedings, 1986. Edited by G. Tinhofer and G. Schmidt. VII, 307 pages. 1987.

Vol. 247: STACS 87. Proceedings, 1987. Edited by F.J. Brandenburg, G. Vidal-Naquet and M. Wirsing. X, 484 pages. 1987.

Vol. 248: Networking in Open Systems. Proceedings, 1986. Edited by G. Müller and R.P. Blanc. VI, 441 pages. 1987.

Vol. 249: TAPSOFT '87. Volume 1. Proceedings, 1987. Edited by H. Ehrig, R. Kowalski, G. Levi and U. Montanari. XIV, 289 pages. 1987.

Vol. 250: TAPSOFT '87. Volume 2. Proceedings, 1987. Edited by H. Ehrig, R. Kowalski, G. Levi and U. Montanari. XIV, 336 pages. 1987.

Vol. 251: V. Akman, Unobstructed Shortest Paths in Polyhedral Environments. VII, 103 pages. 1987.

Vol. 252: VDM '87. VDM – A Formal Method at Work. Proceedings, 1987. Edited by D. Bjørner, C.B. Jones, M. Mac an Airchinnigh and E.J. Neuhold. IX, 422 pages. 1987.

Vol. 253: J.D. Becker, I. Eisele (Eds.), WOPPLOT 86. Parallel Processing: Logic, Organization, and Technology. Proceedings, 1986. V, 226 pages. 1987.

Vol. 254: Petri Nets: Central Models and Their Properties. Advances in Petri Nets 1986, Part I. Proceedings, 1986. Edited by W. Brauer, W. Reisig and G. Rozenberg. X, 480 pages. 1987.

Vol. 255: Petri Nets: Applications and Relationships to Other Models of Concurrency. Advances in Petri Nets 1986, Part II. Proceedings, 1986. Edited by W. Brauer, W. Reisig and G. Rozenberg. X, 516 pages. 1987.

Vol. 256: Rewriting Techniques and Applications. Proceedings, 1987. Edited by P. Lescanne. VI, 285 pages. 1987.

Vol. 257: Database Machine Performance: Modeling Methodologies and Evaluation Strategies. Edited by F. Cesarini and S. Salza. X, 250 pages. 1987.

Vol. 258: PARLE, Parallel Architectures and Languages Europe. Volume I. Proceedings, 1987. Edited by J.W. de Bakker, A.J. Nijman and P.C. Treleaven. XII, 480 pages. 1987.

Vol. 259: PARLE, Parallel Architectures and Languages Europe. Volume II. Proceedings, 1987. Edited by J.W. de Bakker, A.J. Nijman and P.C. Treleaven. XII, 464 pages. 1987.

Vol. 260: D.C. Luckham, F.W. von Henke, B. Krieg-Brückner, O. Owe, ANNA, A Language for Annotating Ada Programs. V, 143 pages. 1987.

Vol. 261: J. Ch. Freytag, Translating Relational Queries into Iterative Programs. XI, 131 pages. 1987.

Vol. 262: A. Burns, A.M. Lister, A.J. Wellings, A Review of Ada Tasking. VIII, 141 pages. 1987.

Vol. 263: A.M. Odlyzko (Ed.), Advances in Cryptology – CRYPTO '86. Proceedings. XI, 489 pages. 1987.

Vol. 264: E. Wada (Ed.), Logic Programming '86. Proceedings, 1986. VI, 179 pages. 1987.

Vol. 265: K.P. Jantke (Ed.), Analogical and Inductive Inference. Proceedings, 1986. VI, 227 pages. 1987.

Vol. 266: G. Rozenberg (Ed.), Advances in Petri Nets 1987. VI, 451 pages. 1987.

Vol. 267: Th. Ottmann (Ed.), Automata, Languages and Programming. Proceedings, 1987. X, 565 pages. 1987.

Vol. 268: P.M. Pardalos, J.B. Rosen, Constrained Global Optimization: Algorithms and Applications. VII, 143 pages. 1987.

Vol. 269: A. Albrecht, H. Jung, K. Mehlhorn (Eds.), Parallel Algorithms and Architectures. Proceedings, 1987. Approx. 205 pages. 1987.

Vol. 270: E. Börger (Ed.), Computation Theory and Logic. IX, 442 pages. 1987.

Vol. 271: D. Snyers, A. Thayse, From Logic Design to Logi Programming. IV, 125 pages. 1987.

Vol. 272: P. Treleaven, M. Vanneschi (Eds.), Future Parallel Compu ters. Proceedings, 1986. V, 492 pages. 1987.

Vol. 273: J.S. Royer, A Connotational Theory of Program Structure V, 186 pages. 1987.

Vol. 274: G. Kahn (Ed.), Functional Programming Languages an Computer Architecture. Proceedings. VI, 470 pages. 1987.

Vol. 275: A.N. Habermann, U. Montanari (Eds.), System Develop ment and Ada. Proceedings, 1986. V, 305 pages. 1987.

Vol. 276: J. Bézivin, J.M. Hullot, P. Cointe, H. Lieberman (Eds. ECOOP '87. European Conference on Object-Oriented Program ming. Proceedings. VI, 273 pages 1987.

Vol. 279: J.H. Fasel, R.M. Keller (Eds.), Graph Reduction. Procee ings, 1986. XVI, 450 pages. 1987.

Vol. 280: M. Venturini Zilli (Ed.), Mathematical Models for the Sema tics of Parallelism. Proceedings, 1986. V, 231 pages. 1987.

Vol. 281: A. Kelemenová, J. Kelemen (Eds.), Trends, Techniques, an Problems in Theoretical Computer Science. Proceedings, 1986. V 213 pages. 1987.

Vol. 282: P. Gorny, M.J. Tauber (Eds.), Visualization in Programmin Proceedings, 1986. VII, 210 pages. 1987.

Vol. 283: D.H. Pitt, A. Poigné, D.E. Rydeheard (Eds.), Catego Theory and Computer Science. Proceedings, 1987. V, 300 page 1987.